What You Always Wanted to Know About Safe Sex and STD's

What You Always Wanted to Know About Safe Sex and STD's

Ronald A. Hagen "Dr. Love"

Writers Club Press
San Jose New York Lincoln Shanghai

What You Always Wanted to Know About Safe Sex and STD's

Writers Club Press
an imprint of iUniverse, Inc.

For information address:
iUniverse, Inc.
5220 S. 16th St., Suite 200
Lincoln, NE 68512
www.iuniverse.com

ISBN: 0-595-20995-5

Printed in the United States of America

Foreword

Sexually Transmitted Diseases & Safe Sex

If you are not concerned about your safety regarding a sexual relationship, then you are not prepared to enter into one. A concerned, intelligent and caring person will insist on safe sex until you know beyond a shadow of a doubt that each of you are free of any STDs and is healthy.

Your decision to enter into a sexual relationship will affect not only yourself, both emotionally and physically, but your partner, your friends and your family.

The two key words to keep in mind in making a decision are respect and responsibility. Respect for yourself and your body and the responsibility for the consequences of your actions.

Until you know for sure that your partner is free of any STD's you must practice safe sex. Abstinence from sexual intercourse is the only fool proof way of avoiding unwanted pregnancies and sexually transmitted diseases. However, the medical field does make a difference between dangerous unprotected sex and the concept of safe sex. Having safe sex is the only way to protect yourself against sexually transmitted diseases, which are very contagious.

Our material discusses in explicate detail sexually transmitted diseases, their symptoms, treatment and cures and how to cope with them. We also talk at length about abstinence and chastity. The book also comprehensively explains the various methods of safe sex, personal hygiene. We explain how to discuss safe sex, STDs and other important issues with your partner. Don't let luck be your co-pilot in a sexual relationship, find out what you need to know when dating now.

Preface

Do you know the difference between sex and safe sex?

In this day and age it is very easy to feel as if something special is missing in one's life. We seem to be busier than ever yet there can be an emptiness deep inside and a craving so strong that we don't know how to define, much less fill.

One way we try to fill that emptiness is by having sex, however

Sex without a loving and safe relationship can lead to a life-time of misery, unwanted pregnancy and deadly diseases.

Young adults who venture into the uncharted and terrifying world of adult dating are filled with anxiety and confusion. After the high school relationships have faded people desire to become involved in a real relationship. However most are confused because they do not know how to socialize and lack the skills and techniques to develop a true and safe relationship. As a result many have turned to alternative and not reliable ways of socializing like personal ads, dating services, chat rooms, and dating phone lines because they aren't sure of their socializing skills and need advice and crave guidelines especially regarding safe sex.

The mission of the book is to provide accurate information and remove the veil of secrecy and the centuries of myths and false beliefs regarding sex and what safe sex really is and to put aside the preconceived notions and misinformation that has been established by the media.

Everyone desires love, sex and a good relationship, however very few understand the techniques, components, and requirements to develop a successful loving relationship and how to avoid unwanted pregnancy and sexually transmitted diseases.

The material in this book is meant to be an informative educational guide to help you achieve that goal. The ultimate goal of dating is to achieve a safe, satisfying, exciting, romantic sexual relationship that will last and be a cornerstone of your life. The unfortunate fact is that today far too many people find themselves chronically dissatisfied with their relationships and sex lives because of unwanted pregnancy and sexually transmitted diseases.

The information in this book is accurate and up-to-date and is written in a sensitive, direct and easy to understand style.

Life is an emotional journey…

…Rescue 911 series can help prepare you and your loved ones for the physical and psychological adventures on that journey!

Introduction

The Rescue 911 series is a collection of information committed to helping individuals make sound, healthy choices regarding their love lives and sexual activities. This book deals with how adults and teens can constructively talk about their sexuality and safe sex. The material reveals the skills and techniques of safe sex and examines and explains some of the various sexually transmitted diseases and the complexities involved in dating like abstinence, safe sex, and the basic fundamentals needed to develop a good relationship using safe sex.

In order to promote a healthy attitude and responsibility, it's essential to maintain an open, communicative attitude about the topic of sex. This book tackles the tough issues regarding sexuality in a respectful but unblinking manner. The human sexual anatomy is discussed at length in a clear, unambiguous fashion. In addition to explaining the biological ticks of the sexual relationship, we discuss some of the psychological ones as well. We give techniques for broaching the topics of safe sex and abstinence. We discuss how dating can be an even more enjoyable experience without the pressures and dangers involved with having sex. We delve deeply into the subject of sexually transmitted diseases, frankly discussing how these ailments are contracted, their symptoms and treatments, as well as who is really at risk. We explain how much protection safe sex actually is and how to properly utilize it.

This may sound like a lot of information to understand, but keep in mind, that this knowledge will benefit both you and your loved ones throughout your lifetimes. Despite the prevalence of sex in our media and culture, many people remain ignorant about fundamental aspects of the sexual relationship or are confused by conflicting reports and information. It's time to finally distinguish the facts from the fiction. An intelligent, open attitude towards sexuality is vital not only for our own happiness, but for that of our children as well. In order to gain the happiness you desire in life, you must develop the proper behavior and thinking patterns that will produce the conditions you desire in an enjoyable and rewarding sexual relationship.

CHAPTER I

It's Your Future Happiness

Teenagers and adults face a difficult battle. A surge of emotions, peer pressures, and hormones tells them to rush into becoming sexually active. This drive is in exact opposition to what these same teenagers are told by their parents, religion or moral code. The teen years can be a tough and dangerous time. Teens go through an emotional struggle—their heart and desires verses their conscious. Decisions made with an immature mindset can spell catastrophe later on in life. In order to make the right decisions it's essential to be honest with one's self and to try to keep an open mind.

When growing up, it is important for teens to seek the acceptance and approval of the adults in their life by adopting their likes and dislikes. However, as they grow it may become difficult to separate their beliefs and values from their parents and friends.

Teens or adults may feel that in order to accepted and liked they have to suppress their own emotions and feelings so that they do not upset others. Many girls will become involved in a controlling relationship because they are willing to sacrifice their true feelings and endure the anxiety they experience in order to be accepted by the one they love and their friends.

People may be ruled by fear that they are not attractive enough, smart enough, talented enough, or important enough for others to accept what they feel and say. It is this emotion that causes many teens to get involved with addictions, self-abuse and self-pity.

These mixed emotions can cause a lot of hurting on the emotional journey of life. We want to be happy so much that it is difficult for us to learn to trust our emotions, instincts, desires, wants and needs because no matter where they turn, either the media or others will try to install their beliefs and values in their life.

What people need to know is that everyone has the same problem especially when it is involving relationships and sex. Everyone wants to have a good relationship and a good sex life, however, very few can talk about it because they feel awkward and it is difficult to be intimate about their feelings.

Millions of Americans find it hard to talk about relationships and sex. Surveys conducted by researchers and institutes strongly support this theory.

Surveys reveal that nearly 9 in 10 men in relationships with women reported serious problems articulating their needs and desires. Nearly half of the women in heterosexual relationships have difficulties articulating their needs and desires when talking to their partners about the relationship or sex. These findings represent all age categories, from teens to seniors.

The surveys reveal that unless people develop the skills to understand then communicate and then cope with the anxiety involved with a relationship and sex, they will continue to have difficulty in resolving problems in their relationships.

It is easier for some to talk about their feelings, however, everyone can learn to overcome their shortcomings and talk intelligently about their feelings and desires. Talking about your needs and sex is doable, you do not need to feel guilty, ashamed, or embarrassed when talking in detail about personal feelings and relationships.

Parents need to be open concerning the topic of sex whether their teens are sexually active or not. Love, sex and relationships can be perilous undertakings for the inexperienced. The information in this book is designed to enable parents and young adults to be able to communicate about the topics that are really important to them. It is possible to protect yourself and your loved ones from AIDS and other STDs, unplanned pregnancies and emotional and physical violence. It all starts with pulling back the veil of secrecy so many people in our society are denied valid and honest information regarding the topic of sex and relationships and the opportunity of simply discussing the topics in an honest and non-critical manner.

Why is it so important to be completely open regarding sexuality? The answer is that unfortunately, all teens are significantly at risk. No matter how good a person is, one misguided or careless sexual encounter can create any number of disastrous results. Saying, "It won't happen to my child," doesn't make it so.

In today's world it has become more difficult for people to become properly prepared for the sexual and emotional journey that they are going to undertake during their lifetime. When people are young they are naturally very involved exploring and defining their own identities while at the same time trying to assert their independence for the first time. Although this is a normal evolutionary process for teenagers, it often creates power struggles and tensions in the parent / child relationship. Unfortunately, no matter how thoughtful a parent is, it is very difficult at times to communicate effectively and to have the child benefit from the parent's experiences and knowledge.

Our young people are especially vulnerable emotionally and physically to the aftermath of an unprepared or premature sexual encounter. Many teenagers are not properly protected against undesired pregnancies, disease and exploitation.

One of the main hurdles for parents to overcome in trying to communicate with their teens is the attitude that, "This doesn't happen to me and my friends, we're above this, that's only what you see on TV." Sadly, most people learn too soon in life that terrible things do happen to every one, from all classes, all economic and educational backgrounds. No matter where you live or work, you and your teenagers are exposed to tremendous temptations, exploitations and risks.

Both for teenagers and adults, the consequences of indiscriminate, early sexual encounters leaves them exposed to tremendous sexual torment, anxiety and violence unprepared and unplanned pregnancies and the life threatening sexually transmitted diseases.

Although tempting, trying to "turn off" the world is not a viable option. Sometimes parents can become overprotective and shelter their teens too much. Although this may prove to be a solution for a few years, this tactic can ultimately have deeply negative results. Raising teens in a social / sexual vacuum does not prepare them for the real world. When they inevitably have to leave that vacuum, they may find themselves woefully ill equipped to deal with the temptations and pitfalls of adult sexuality.

One of the main major hurdles that parents face with their teens today is addressing the issue of sex in the first place. For generations, centuries really, a veil of secrecy has covered the topic of sexuality and any activity associated with it. As a result, because of cultural backgrounds, religious beliefs and even governmental mandates, we have fostered a system where many people grow up in almost complete ignorance of sex and relationships.

Simply put, the institutions of today's society aren't doing a very good job of teaching the facts. We cannot rely on our schools to impart the proper knowledge and protect our children. Although there are sex education courses given in class, they teach little more than basic anatomy and facts about the birth process. Rarely if ever do they tackle the really tough subjects of sexual activity such as how to establish values, how to build the fundamental elements necessary for a good relationship, what the benefits and drawbacks are of intimacy and pleasure or how to emotionally face that fateful day when a love affair ends. As our society demonstrates constantly, the emotional scars of bad sexual relationships run deep and sometimes never fully heal.

It's a huge mistake to subscribe to the quicksand psychology that if parents and role models preach abstinence and chastity that is all that is necessary. Parents should encourage their children to delay sexual activity, but this doesn't mean that parents should make sexuality a taboo subject. If parents haven't prepared their children, they may be setting them up for calamity latter on. The results of sexual ignorance are just as disastrous for someone at age 23 as they are for someone at 14 or 15. This is clearly shown in the results of numerous research studies, interviews and surveys. Charts or graphs aren't even necessary to prove this point. All most Americans have to do is to look at a weekly magazine or daily newspaper to see the tremendous physical and emotional scars that many bear as a result of terrible sexual relationships. It is not enough to simply postpone going into a relationship. Preparation, information and honesty are needed in order to protect one's self.

At times it seems that too much information has been made available for people to still be irresponsible about sex, and yet it happens constantly. Teenagers have to be made to understand that if someone isn't concerned about their safety regarding a sexual relationship, then they shouldn't enter into one. Only a concerned, intelligent, caring person will insist on safe sex . Self -respect is a slippery topic in regards to teens, and all too often it's determined largely by the view of their peer group. Teens need to be taught that in order for others to respect you, you must respect yourself first. Teenagers need to make it a matter of personal pride that they respect themselves too much to risk their futures or their lives on ill planned, indiscriminate sexual encounters.

In addition, teens must be taught to find a value in people, not in things that people possess. All too often teenagers end up with a twisted perception of affection, equating money, fame or sexual prowess with success in dating and relationships. If left unchecked, such an attitude can form the template of their adult personalities. The real truth is that money, fame and power play a very minor role in a good sexual relationship, and without the right components it's impossible to build a loving, long term connection.

Teens must learn that sex is but a part of a larger experience in life. One of the major factors governing the outcome of a person's life is how they handle their sexual activities. It's essential to always consider the potential life long effects of having sex. There always looms the ominous potential of having an unwanted pregnancy or contracting a painful or even life threatening STD.

No single sex act, no matter how pleasurable, is worth a lifetime of discomfort and pain.

There are thousands of wrong reasons for entering into a sexual relationship. Peer pressure, curiosity, jealousy, trying to impress someone, trying to prove maturity are among the most common. One of the most prevalent and saddest reasons that teens have sex is to feel love, or to attempt to make others love them. However, the only real reason to have a sexual relationship is when two mature, consenting people that are emotionally, mentally, and physically prepared and have had the time to thoroughly think about what they are doing and feel comfortable about their decisions to have a sexual relationship.

Cardinal Rule

Never confuse sex with love. Having sex does not create love.

The most important decision in your lifetime is choosing the right mate and relationship because it will account for the majority of the happiness or misery that you will experience in your future.

Cardinal Rule

> **Problems are not solved by having sex.**
> **Sadness and low self-esteem are a cause of sex,**
> **and sex is a cause of sadness and low self-esteem.**

It is unfortunate, but sexual relationships can present us with enormous problems. A good relationship can be the most wondrous, beautiful, satisfying, rewarding facet of one's life. A poor or bad sexual relationship can be terrifying, emotionally agonizing and in some cases, deadly. It's vital for parents to learn to be understanding and sensitive and for teenagers not to allow their hormones to run rampant and let the mass media dictate their guidelines and values.

One should never let luck be their co-pilot in a sexual relationship.

Sexual Control

The mission of this book is to provide you with enough knowledge and concern to give you a moral backbone and enable you to make the right decision concerning your sexual activity. In the real world most teens are preoccupied with the idea of dating and sex. Teenagers natural curiosity is fed by a constant barrage of sexually suggestive and explicit messages from the media. Like it or not—sex and sexual activity are a part of our every day life and permeate nearly every layer of our society. Whether you approve or disapprove, understand or don't understand, we are confronted with sexual choices every day of our lives. The media has inundated us with information that causes many confusion and anxiety and ultimately ends up negatively influencing our attitudes and behavior

Despite this proliferation of sexually charged material, our society still remains rather nervous towards the subject. The veil of secrecy about sexuality and sexual relationships remains intact even today, leaving both the young and old on their own to understand and explain sexuality. As a result, dangerous ideas and beliefs have been passed on from generation to generation for decades, perhaps even centuries. People learn more regarding sex and sexual activity from uninformed peers and the advertising media than they do from their parents, school or church. In today's society we are experiencing so many poor, bad or failed relationships and an increase in sexually transmitted diseases because people have come to accept and believe these myths.

CHAPTER II

The New Pathway

Why Teens and Parents Must Communicate

Before we can discuss such things as abstinence, safe sex and sexual health we need to explain why it is important for parents and teens to communicate, along with providing techniques that promote trust and parent / child closeness.

Few teenagers are mature or emotionally conditioned enough to make them capable of safely managing their sex lives. Therefore responsible and knowledgeable parents need to do whatever is necessary to help guide their teenagers. This is easier said than done, as many parents often need to come to terms with the fact that their teens need their help in the first place.

All teenagers are looking for answers of one sort or another. Many times they are left to draw upon their own experiences and peers to get answers on sex and safe sex. This is an extremely dangerous route because frequently the answers they get are not complete or are just blatantly incorrect. Parents need to be ready to answer their children's questions in a straight forward manner and *not put it off.*. Otherwise they will get the answers from somebody else who might provide bad information or mess with their emotions or morals.

Most generation-Xers discover that hanging out with high school and college pals won't prepare them for the world of no-rules sex and romance.

A free flow of communication is essential to create a solid bond between parents and their teens. Everything that is discussed in this book and all of the information offered will be useless unless one is able to discuss their feelings and thoughts honestly. It's not enough just to speak honestly however. In order to truly succeed as a great communicator one must make their ears honest as well. It's essential for parents to always realize that communication is a two way street, and that stopping to listen often can be more effective than any advice or platitudes that one has to offer.

Cardinal Rule

Preventive maintenance is necessary to help teenagers through difficult times. Parents must learn to converse easily with their teens in order to help them understand the dangers of being sexually active. Most teens really want the help and assurance, but are too nervous or embarrassed to ask. Learning to talk about sex with your daughter or son can be hard, but it has never been more important.

Learn to Communicate Honestly

Sometimes the truth hurts, but there are ways to improve your sex-talk skills without hurting the other person or causing bad feelings. You never want to clause an argument because that will only lead to more anxiety and arguments.

The following are simple ways to improve your relationship talk skills:

1. Never leave your sexual wishes and desires to guesswork, learn to communicate them clearly and honestly.
2. Talk to your partner as you would your best friend, learn to confine your real feelings like you would to a friend.

3. When you ask a question, give your partner a chance to answer.

4. Always listen to what he or she is saying with an open mind and be realistic about your decisions. If you cannot agree about something, then try to find a middle ground. Learning to compromise is the secret to eliminating frustration and building a good relationship.

5. If your partner is doing something that pleases you then tell him or her. This is called positive reinforcement. And when a person learns that they are pleasing another person their ego is increased and they will want to please you in the future again and again.

6. Make specific concrete request, such as, "please kiss me, hug me, hold me". A request will more likely give you the desired result then when you express a vague wish like, let's be more romantic".

7. Talk honestly and intimately about sex afterwards, about what he or she did that pleased you, always state your preferences in a positive manner, this will get much better results because you will reinforce a positive feeling. For example, "I like it when you touch me like this" or "I like it when you do this to me", this sounds much better and will get the response you want. When you say something like "you don't do this right, or I don't' like this", you will evoke a hurt feeling and will not get the results that you desire.

8. Never ask your partner to do something that they are not emotionally or mentally capable of doing.

9. Do not ask a question that does not have a realistic or practical answer.

10. Take turns talking about topics that the other person is interested in.

11. Do not get into heated arguments regarding topics that cannot be resolved, like religion, family, politics, careers, or desires this will only evoke long-term anxiety and hurt feelings.

12. Learn to listen to the other person with respect and empathy for their feelings and viewpoints. You may not agree with them, but you do need to understand why they feel the way they do.

13. Learn to laugh at small problems, small faults, minor mistakes, treat your partner like you would your best friend and forgive or overlook innocent mistakes or faults.

14. Never put pressure on your partner to make a decision that they're not ready to make. This could cause resentment or an argument.

15. Be optimistic when your partner is trying to explain something it will make understanding and if necessary forgiving much easier.

16. Remember that many kinds of questions have no right or wrong answer, and no "yes" or "no" answer.

17. Patience and cooperation are necessary to finding the solution to a problem, because sometimes the solution is not obvious or simple and many times there is no quick fix.

18. In order for your relationship to have staying power you must realize, you will never always have the same likes and dislikes. Therefore be honest in expressing your feelings so that the other person does not misunderstand and have a false impression of what you like or don't like. Candor is the key to expressing your likes and dislikes.

19. Don't belittle your partner's wants or desires, learn to show compassion.

20. Learn to establish ground rules regarding the sensitive topics that you will discuss with your partner.

21. When you're wrong learn to say "I'm sorry" sincerely. Do not create a dispute because you cannot say "I'm sorry".

22. Learn to express your feelings by saying, "I love you" and "I care about you". Everyone needs to hear this to reinforce the relationship.

23. Never judge a person based on their actions only, always find out the reason or logic behind the action.

24. Speak with respect to your partner otherwise they may feel threatened and resent talking to you.

25. Whenever someone asks you something that is very personal and you don't want to answer the question, asked them why they need to know? Their reason may help you with your answer.

26. Never verbally attack your mate because they will be unwilling to open up about themselves and may resent what your saying. If they are doing something that annoys you and you want to change their behavior make a positive suggestion of how they could improve the relationship.

27. If you have a pessimistic outlook regarding what your mate is telling you then the conversation will become destined to have a self-fulfilling negative outcome.

28. Do not repudiate another person's values without understanding their feelings, then try to embrace the difference or find a middle ground to compromise.

29. Remember when you're angry that silence may be the best form of communication.

30. If you have a quarrel with your partner try not to involve past events or people, but focus on solving the present issues.

31. Learning to understand and compromise is the secret to a long-term relationship.

Falling in love is easy, staying in love and having a good relationship takes effort.

The most important guideline to good communication is to establish some ground rules regarding your discussion. This will enable you to get your point across without trampling your partners feelings under foot in the process. The main areas that should be observed regarding ground rules are as follows:

1. Never argue or belittle the other person in front of friends, family or in public.

2. Learn to discuss problems and tell your true feelings, even if it's easier for you to lie.

3. Have empathy for the other persons feelings and needs. Don't belittle their wants and desires. Don't dismiss their questions or requests (many times parents assume that their teen is already aware of something, when in reality they're not).

4. Try to never fight or argue when you're angry or upset. Emotions will run rampant and feelings will be severely hurt, many times creating a barrier to communication.

5. Establish some quiet time when you can sit down with the other person and discuss their questions and concerns.

6. Keep a regular channel of communication open. Always let them know that you are there to listen.

7. Don't let friends or neighbors set your standards or opinions.

8. If you have difficulty explaining something because it is an emotional topic you should write it in a note and give the note to the other person. This may prevent heated disagreements.

Establishing some ground rules is very important because it enables families to maintain order in their discussions while promoting self-respect in their children. These aren't rules for parents alone to obey, it's essential for teens to adopt them as well. In this way both parent and child can feel confident and safe when dealing with each other.

How to Communicate With Your Teen Regarding Emotions, Chastity, Pregnancy, and STDs

A new approach to safe sex is needed to change the growing trends of unwanted pregnancies, increasing levels of STDs and abortions. It becomes clear that the traditional approach to solving these problems has not been effective. Information is the key – only by learning the truth about safe sex can one control their future.

This book does not discuss the morality of whether or not one should engage in a sexual relationship outside of marriage. That is a question that has to be answered on an individual basis. It's a decision that can't be made lightly. It's essential for one to openly and honestly examine their own moral, cultural and religious values before choosing whether or not to become sexually active. A large part of making that decision is gaining an intelligent understanding of what exactly safe sex is and how it can be implemented in a relationship.

Categories of safe sex:

1. Abstinence and chastity
2. Sexual history and medical exams
3. Safe sex procedures

It's essential that parents explain to their children what they'll need to know when they eventually do enter into a sexual relationship. First and foremost, teens need to be taught to understand STDs, and to realize the need to talk to their potential partner about them *BEFORE* they have any sort of intimate contact. Parents must stress to their teens the importance of being honest with their partners about their own health as well. Telling a prospective partner about one's medical history can be difficult, but it's an important responsibility. Teens need to understand that patience is a virtue in relationships. One must allow enough time to get to know their partner before becoming intimate with that person. There are no short cuts for gaining trust. Even if a teen is still years away from sexual activity, it's important for them to understand how to properly communicate about sexual health and medical histories for when that time inevitably comes.

When Do You Discuss STDs or Medical Histories With Your Partner?

It's essential to broach the topic of medical histories and sexual health before any sort of intimacy happens in a relationship. All too often people wait until they have become engaged in a passionate session to tell their partner about their STD. This is a thoughtless tactic that can very often lead to hurt feelings or a complete break up. It's best for one to stay relaxed and confident and to explain to their partner in a quiet manner what has been involved with their medical history or sexual health.

Even if sexual contact has already occurred, it's still never too late to have this discussion.

Where Do You Want to Talk to Your Partner About Your Medical History or STD?

Any sensitive discussions should occur someplace that is secure, private and safe. It's important for both partners in the relationship to feel as comfortable as possible. It's a mistake to have such a talk in a public place. One should never have this discussion on the phone or over a computer as this is immensely impersonal and likely to cause hurt feelings.

What Do You Confide In Your Partner?

When a person wants to discuss their medical history or sexually transmitted disease with a partner, it always helps to express respect and trust before the discussion even begins. Once the conversation has started, it's important to remain positive and open to questions and concerns. There are certain questions that must be answered before any sexual contact occurs. It's vital to find out if both partners have always used proper protection in prior relationships (such as a condom). Discussing past sex partners is important as well, but is a topic that must be handled sensitively and non-critically.

As many STDs have an incubation period of months, it might not be obviously apparent that a person is infected. Current medical exams and blood work are the only truly reliable ways of determining whether or not an STD is present, so both partners should get a check up if they've been sexually active previously. If an STD is involved in either partner's health profile, it needs to be frankly discussed. Treatments and protective measures need to be determined before the relationship can proceed any further.

It's important to stay positive. Getting involved with issues of blame, guilt or fault finding accomplishes nothing and can only lead to anger or depression. Talking about sexual health can be uncomfortable at first, but it ultimately creates more trust and intimacy in a relationship when handled in a thoughtful manner.

It takes only one unprotected encounter to contract a sexually transmitted disease. No single sex act is worth a lifetime of discomfort or your life itself. Always be concerned enough to ask about a partner's medical history.

Cardinal Rule

> A loving relationship is a two-way street.
> Remember no one is without fault. Understanding and
> compromise is the key to unlocking happiness.

A sexual relationship is as much an emotional state of mind as a physical relationship. The thoughts of another, the anticipation of an affair, the planning of a romantic interlude, a loving, note, a caring whisper in the ear, a special look or gesture, a phone call, a thoughtful act, words of praise or encouragement, a hug, a tender touch, sharing a special moment together, having that someone special near you, words of understanding, a helping hand, trust, loyalty, are all part of a good sexual relationship, and may bring the greatest pleasures and create the strongest bond, if done at the proper time and when you are prepared.

In order to establish a good sexual relationship, both parties must be emotionally mature and emotionally prepared and have a good attitude toward sex. Without these key elements no physical stimulation, no physical enticements will ever result in achieving a truly wonderful, satisfying and pleasurable sexual relationship by themselves. It is only in concert with one's mental and emotional state that one can truly experience the ultimate sexual relationship.

Thus the key to developing a good sexual relationship is to have good communication between the partners and to make sure that they are both emotionally prepared to develop a pleasurable and satisfying sexual relationship. Without this mutual understanding and consent the relationship will never be able to obtain its full goals and develop a sound foundation for a caring long term, relationship.

The first major step in developing a good sexual relationship is to understand you cannot control the relationship. You cannot control another's feelings. You may try, however, history shows that this never succeeds in the long run. Trying to control the other individual's feelings many times will push that person away from you and destroy whatever feelings you have for each other. The two key things is developing a good sexual relationship is understanding and using the key elements of a sexual relationship and consent by the individuals. Therefore, in developing a good relationship you must learn to adjust and understand. You must have empathy for the other person's feelings and needs. Find out what will make them fulfilled and happy, then incorporate these elements into your relationships. A relationship is a unique bond between two individuals that is held together by intimacy and honesty. The intimacy and honesty that creates the unity of a relationship.

The intimacy and honesty allows people to become closer and closer until that bond enables the person to not only grow within themselves, but support and help the other person grow in the relationship as well. Honest communication is the key to developing a good relationship; it is the key to understanding chastity. Honestly expressing yourself is the key to control STD's and it is the major component which you have control over in a relationship. Without honest communication you will never establish trust in your relationship. Honesty and trust are the cornerstones of a solid relationship. Without trust in a relationship you will never be able to discuss and practice chastity, abstinence and safe sex.

CHAPTER III

Chastity and Abstinence

Do you know the difference between sex, love and a relationship? Having a sexual relationship is one of the most important voluntary choices a person can make. It will affect you emotionally and physically. If you chose not to be sexually active and want to protect yourself, then abstinence is the proper decision for you.

Sexual thoughts and feelings are normal, everyone has them. Sexual desires go along with physical and emotional development, so do not be embarrassed or nervous by them. Following abstinence does not mean that you do not believe in kissing, necking, petting, stroking or that you have to stay away completely from the opposite sex. It refers to abstaining from sexual intercourse, usually until marriage. Some people feel that avoiding temptation is necessary to avoid physical intimacy all together. In general, if you are practicing abstinence it is unwise to get into a passionate situation where you're going to be tempted to fulfill your urges. Still it is important to understand that these urges and desires are normal and good.

Abstinence has many rewards. Being a virgin is something to be proud of. Chastity is a good basis for self esteem. It allows you to be free of any worry or guilt. It means that you will be safe from all sexually transmitted diseases. It means that you have given yourself enough time to make sure you are ready for the responsibilities that go along with a sexual relationship. Abstinence allows a partner to be more open and honest.

Cardinal Rule

> Safe sex is *not* 100% effective, only chastity is 1*00*% protection for your most precious gift.

The key to developing a good relationship is to be patient. Going too fast emotionally and physically can damage the sexual relationship. One must be emotionally as well as physically prepared for the relationship. One must feel comfortable and consent to the relationship. Remember, physical sex does not make a sexual relationship. You must be truly ready and prepared to make all the commitments that we have been discussing in this book

Sex can cause a lot of pain and sadness when people think sex is love. Having sex does not create love, but having sex without love at the wrong time, without the proper intentions or relationship can cause a variety of negative feelings and leave one vulnerable to STD's and unwanted pregnancies.

You must learn to take control of your body and life—learn so say "**no**" to premarital sex.

Keeping a relationship going is hard work and do not rely upon sex otherwise you will be disappointed.

Sex can fool you for a while and lead you into dating or marrying the wrong person. Sex can create a strong emotional bond and make you believe that you are in love and have a whole relationship. Your judgment can become clouded, leading you to a commitment that ultimately isn't right for you. When the sex and romance fade and you come to realize that there are no lasting commitments, values or plans, only terrible frustration is left along with regret and sadness.

Learning to say "no" to unplanned sex will make you a happier person. People believe that their dreams will come true when they have sex with that special person, but usually if you rush your relationship and blindly follow your passion, it is not your dreams that come true but your nightmares as you watch your relationship crumble and loneliness and sadness take over.

Do not follow the path of regret. It is not enough for people to feel passion in a heavy caressing and kissing session and to express words of endearment. It must be true feelings. People often say words of endearment during a hormonal moment, it is commonly called "pillow talk". If you try to push a relationship, you may end up destroying the relationship because you are moving too suddenly for your partner. You may end up having feelings of guilt or of being used. You may end up emotionally scarred because the words of endearment that were said during the moment of passion turned out to be false. Frustration, anxiety and hatred can set in very quickly in place of what you though was love.

Learn to be mature, allow love and relationships to grow naturally. Learning to say "no" at the proper time can show how highly you feel about yourself and others and what a high value you place on your commitment and sexuality. You can feel proud that you have no regrets and have avoided frustrations, sadness and STD's.

Both partners should take their time to really get to know the other partner's plans, likes, desires, needs, feelings and morals. When it feels natural and right, you will know it. When it is time to make a real conscientious commitment you will feel good about the decision.

Give love and happiness time to mature and develop into a whole relationship. Keep a good reputation, stay healthy, have no regrets, avoid sadness, frustration and unwanted pregnancies, guilt and disappointment by following chastity and saying "no".

The status of one's virginity is a delicate topic that must be discussed in a meaningful way in order not to cause problems in the development of a sexual relationship. To wait to discuss one's sexual preferences and plans until one is in the midst of a steamy, passionate caressing session could cause some undesirable effects. One partner may feel rebutted by the other if they themselves are not a virgin. There may be a belief by one partner that the other is using their virginity as an excuse to not become involved in a deeper relationship.

Saying that one is a virgin at the inappropriate time will add to the confusion of a blossoming relationship. Before a developing love affair becomes too intense, discuss your feelings openly. Tell the other person what your true attitudes are towards sex and be direct in communicating to your partner what is agreeable to you. In this manner you can gain respect and admiration from your partner and the two of you can then work on the same level towards a meaningful and rewarding relationship. There is a wonderful and delightful world of sexual sensations and pleasures that can be enjoyed without having sexual intercourse. Until you are ready to make that commitment, you should be comfortable in the relationship that you are developing because you know what goals you want to obtain.

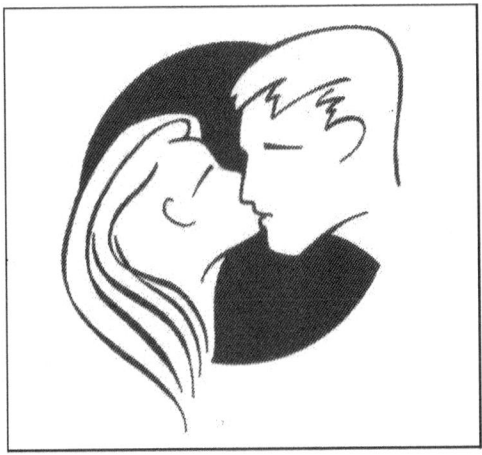

CHAPTER IV

Safe Sex Procedures

Sex is a good and natural process, a wonderful part of a relationship and is necessary for procreation. However, too much information has been made available for you to be irresponsible about sex. If you are not concerned about your safety regarding a sexual relationship, then you are not prepared to enter into one. A concerned, intelligent and caring person will insist on safe sex until you known beyond a doubt that each of your are free from any STDs and healthy.

Safer sex does not mean eliminating sex from your life. It does mean being smart and staying healthy. It means self-respect and respect for your partner—talking about sex, knowing how to protect yourself, and taking precautions every time. Safer sex means enjoying sex without giving or getting sexually transmitted diseases. It is what you do, not who you are, that creates a risk for sexually transmitted diseases—and you can protect yourself by the precautions you take.

Your decision to enter into a sexual relationship will affect not only yourself, but potentially your partner, your friends and your family as well. The two key words to keep in mind when making a decision are "respect" and "responsibility." Respect yourself and your body, and take responsibility for your own actions.

There are thousands of wrong reasons for entering into a sexual relationship. However, as we have discussed and try to convey in this book, you must be both emotionally and physically prepared. Think things through clearly, so that you don't feel uncomfortable and that when you get into a sexual relationship, it will be a good experience that will make you feel happy and whole. You must consider the potential life-long effects of having sex.

Physical intimacy can be a warm, caring, exciting experience. It also requires thought, planning, and responsibility. Choosing to be sexually active requires we take precautions to protect ourselves and our partners from sexually transmitted diseases(STDs). It is important to make sexual intimacy as enjoyable and safe as possible.

Many people believe that if a person wants answers to their questions on sex, they can go to their parents, family doctor or teacher. However, the reality is that most people feel uncomfortable discussing the subject. Children rarely seek answers from their parents, the school system rarely has good programs on sexual education, and many churches rely upon the family and the parents for sexual education. As a result of this veil of secrecy, it is clear form many of the surveys and studies that have been done in the past 10 years, including the Kinsey Institute and Roper National Sex Knowledge Test, demonstrate that the vast majority of people of both sexes and all ages are either unaware or improperly informed regarding sexual relationships and especially sexually transmitted diseases, their causes, symptom and cures. This section is to furnish the information that is so overwhelmingly needed in our society today but is not readily available to those seeking answers to the questions and assistance in developing the most important decision in their life. Choosing the right partner and forming a long term relationship, is the most important decision one will make in their lifetime because it will determine 90% of the happiness or misery that they will experience during that lifetime.

Cardinal Rule

Safe sex is important to a relationship because it creates confidence and trust between the partners by reaffirming each other's value of self.

Abstinence from sexual intercourse is the only foolproof way of having safe sex regarding unwanted pregnancies and sexually transmitted diseases. However, the medical field does make a difference between dangerous unprotected sex and the concept of safe sex. Having safe sex is the only way to protect yourself against sexually transmitted diseases, which are very contagious. You cannot tell if a person has a STD by looks: in fact, many people that are infected look and feel fine and appear healthy. The infected person may be unaware that they are infected, or ashamed or angry that they are infected and will not tell anyone. Never even take it for granted, you must be responsible, use your head, not your heart until you are certain that your new partner is not infected. Having sexual intercourse even one time with someone who is infected can expose a person to sexually transmitted disease and aids. These diseases can cause infertility, sterility, genital pain and irritation, nervous disorders, and even death. STDs can be spread through almost any body fluid, therefore, vaginal, oral and anal sex can cause the spread and infection of an STD.

Cardinal Rule

When you become involved with a new lover, you must always practice safe sex until both of you have had a complete medical exam and blood tests for STDs. As a show of good faith show your test results and make sure you see your partner' results. *Never* take someone's verbal statement of good health. If your lover refuses to show their test results, immediately stop the relationship.

Simple and Safe

STDs are spread by infectious microorganisms such as bacteria, viruses, and parasites moving from one person to another. Different microorganisms are spread in different ways. Most travel only in certain body fluids like blood, semen, and vaginal secretions. Some sexually related microorganisms can be transmitted in saliva, and a few are spread by direct skin-to-skin contact. Making sexual intimacy as enjoyable and safe as possible means knowing what kinds of intimate contact transmit various STDs. Protecting yourself means choosing only safer sex practices, suing latex barriers against STDs correctly and consistently, or not having sex. You do not have to have sex with a lot of people to get STDs. Your chance of acquiring STDs increases when you have unprotected sex, no matter how many partners you have. **Always take precautions whenever you have sex.**

Condoms, unfortunately, have not traditionally had a good position in our society. They were "those things" you used to guard against pregnancy. However, because of the increased public awareness of sexually transmitted diseases in general and AIDS in particular, they are now in style and the safest and most preferred way to have safe sex.

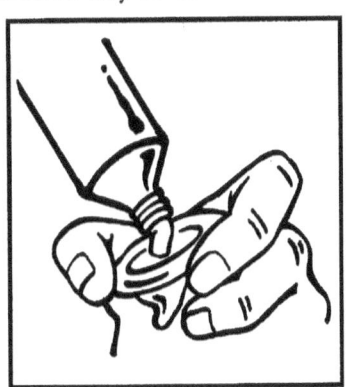

Condoms, when used in conjunction with a spermicide, or spermicide cream, are extremely effective in not only preventing unwanted pregnancies, but in protection from unwanted sexually transmitted diseases and

Aids. There procure are widely available and in some cases freely given out. There is no reason for anyone to have unprotected sex.

A large number of medical studies have shown that latex condoms, especially if coupled with a spermicide, can dramatically reduce the chances of becoming infected with an STD. This is not to say that condoms are guaranteed to be 100% effective. They cannot completely eliminate the risk of contracting an STD or of preventing a pregnancy. Nevertheless they are the recommended and the preferred method. These products are widely available, and in some cases freely given out. There is no reason for anyone to have unprotected sex.

The proper technique to use spermicide with a latex condom.

The most important rule regarding condoms is to put the condom on before the penis comes in contact with the vagina. Most people don't realize that the penis will extrude small amounts of sperm and fluid before the full fledged ejaculation takes place. This is sufficient to cause both pregnancy and the contraction of a sexually transmitted disease. Place the correct side of the condom against the head of the penis and unroll it all the way down to the base of the penis (if the condom does not unroll easily, you have it backwards). Pinch the tip of the condom as you roll it on, so that there is some empty space at the end, preferably one half of an inch. Try not to leave a bubble of air at the tip as this may cause the condom to slip or burst.

The condom is very thin and is designed for protection and to give as much sensitivity as possible to both partners. The best way to penetrate the woman is to wait until she is well lubricated, or use a water-based lubricant. A non-lubricated vagina is more likely to tear the condom. Sometimes penetration with a dry condom or dry penis can be irritable and painful for the woman. After intercourse, always remove the condom and avoid spillage of its contents. Check the condom for leaks and discard it. **Never reuse a condom under any circumstances.** Some people believe that they can wash a condom and reuse it. This is unsanitary and may help to promote the very diseases the condom was designed to protect against.

Proper technique to put on a latex condom

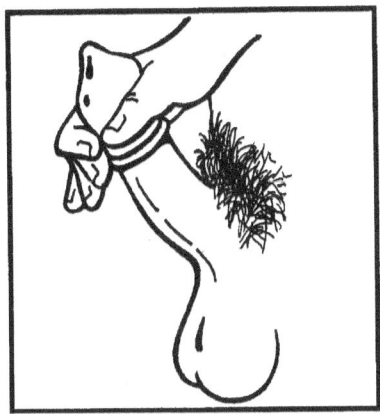

If you discover a leak, have your partner immediately apply spermicide to her vagina without delay. Do a proper washing. Medical studies have shown that even in the case of some sexually transmitted diseases, if the area is completely flushed out and washed with soap, it will destroy or remove the STD. If a condom breaks while being used to guard against pregnancy, then the woman should consult with her physician as soon as possible. You may be able to get a morning after pill, which can reduce the chances of getting pregnant if taken within 72 hours of intercourse.

Special notes regarding condoms:

Avoid using condoms that are more than two years old. It may have deteriorated and be more prone to breakage. Store condoms in a dry place away from heat and light. Unfortunately, many people are used to carrying condoms in a purse or wallet. These are bad places to keep them for any long period of time.

Never, under any circumstances, use petroleum based lubricants, like Vaseline, with a condom. Never use vaginal medications, including Monistat, Premarin, Estrace, Vagisil or any other feminine product. These products have a chemical in them that will cause the latex condom to deteriorate, allowing the passage of sperm and microscopic organisms. In the book Love, Sex & Relationships I discuss some exciting and exotic ways to put on condoms so that it can be a part of the foreplay and pleasure for both the man and the woman. Recently, researchers have developed a female product that serves as a condom. However, medical studies have shown that this device is not as trustworthy as a traditional, male worn condom. The female condom has a tendency to be pushed or moved out of place prematurely and, therefore, does not offer the protection that the traditional male condom offers.

How to Use a Condom Guide
Department of Health and Human Services, Food and Drug Administration

1. Follow these guidelines:
2. Use a new condom for every act of intercourse.
3. If the penis is uncircumcised, pull the foreskin back before putting the condom on.
4. Put the condom on after the penis is erect (hard) and before any contact is made between the penis and any part of the partner's body.
5. If using a spermicide, put some inside the condom tip.
6. If the condom does not have a reservoir tip, pinch the tip enough to leave a half-inch space for semen to collect.
7. While pinching the half-inch tip, place the condom against the penis and unroll it all the way to the base. Put more spermicide or lubricant on the outside.

8. If you feel a condom break while you are having sex, stop immediately and pull out. Do not continue until you have put on a new condom and used more spermicide.

9. After ejaculation and before the penis gets soft, grip the rim of the condom and carefully withdraw from your partner.

10. To remove the condom from the penis, pull it off gently, being careful semen doesn't spill out.

11. Wrap the used condom in a tissue and throw it in the trash where others won't handle it. Because condoms may cause problems in sewers, don't flush them down the toilet. Afterwards, wash your hands with soap and water.

Beware of drugs and alcohol! **They can affect your judgment**, so you may forget to use a condom. They may even affect your ability to use a condom properly.

One final note: Do not become confused by the word contraceptive. Many contraceptives are devices that are effective only in preventing pregnancies and offer absolutely NO protection against AIDS or other sexually transmitted diseases. For example, diaphragms, cervical caps and contraceptive sponges all prevent pregnancy, but do little to guard against disease. The only recommended protection for both unwanted pregnancies and sexually transmitted diseases is the traditional male worn condom.

Practicing safer sex means engaging in sexual intercourse that can potentially be dangerous. However, you can drastically reduce the risk by using the proper precautions until you and your partner have had an opportunity to have a complete medical examination and know for sure that you are healthy and STD free. This will allow you to have unprotected sex if you are not concerned about the pregnancy aspect. Safer sex allows you to enjoy sexual contact without acquiring sexually transmitted diseases.

You should always use a latex condom plus spermicide containing nonoxynol-9 when having sexual intercourse. When you start a new sexual relationship, chose your partner wisely, share sexual and medical histories and have the appropriate medical examinations done before ever having any sexual contact without a latex condom. STDs are transmitted through blood and certain other bodily fluids such as amniotic fluid, pericardial fluid, peritoneal fluid, pleural fluid, synovial fluid, cerebrospinal fluid, semen, vaginal secretions).

The following chart can be used as a guide:

RISK AND PREVENTION CHART

Amount of Activity	Amount of Risk	Precautions to Take
Abstinence	**NO RISK**	No precautions necessary
Sex with a single partne7r	**LOW RISK** If you have sex with only one person who also has had no other sex partner and neither of you has an STD, you have practically no risk of being infected.	**Use condoms during sex.** Wearing condoms are the most effective preventative measure sex partners can take. Men should wear condoms and women should insist male partners use them. Condoms are not fool proof, but they are usually effective.
Sex with a few people you know well	**SOME RISK** If you have sex with a few people you know well, your risk increases. You have some control over risk by choosing partners carefully.	Use condoms during sex. Use spermicidal. Wash after sex. Urinate after sex.
Your partner has sex with others.	**INCREASED RISK** If you have sex with only one person but your partner has sex with others, your risk increases. That is because you have no control over your partner's partners.	Use condoms during sex. Use spermicidal. Wash after sex. Urinate after sex.
Sex with many partners	**HIGH RISK** If you have sex with many people – particularly people you do not know well, you are at high risk of getting an STD.	Use condoms during sex. Use spermicidal. Wash after sex. Urinate after sex.

Cardinal Rule

Coitus interruptus—withdrawal of the penis from the vagina just before ejaculation is *NOT* an effective form of birth control and offers NO protection against STDs.

No matter how exciting a sex act is, it takes only one unprotected encounter to contract a sexually transmitted disease. No single sex act, no matter how pleasurable, is worth a lifetime of pain and discomfort.

Every situation and relationship is unique. Be honest and practice what you say, let your partner know your concerns. Emphasize that you care and want to protect both of you, sex is so much more fun when you have the peace of mind because you and your partner used proper protection and safe sex methods.

Safer sex can greatly reduce your chances of getting an STD, but sometimes infection may still occur. If you think you have been exposed to an STD, it is important to be examined, tested, and treated as soon as possible. Even if you have no symptoms now, an STD could cause serious health risks and problems for you and your partner later. People sometimes feel ashamed or guilty about STDs. Don't let your feelings stop you from getting help, or from letting your partner(s) get help. Medically effective, non-judgmental treatment and information (often free, or at low cost) is available from:

1. College/university health services
2. Public health departments or community STD clinics
3. Skilled private physicians

Condoms

Throughout the book we refer to condoms or latex condoms. Although there are a variety of styles and materials, the ONLY condom that we refer to is a latex condom. The preferred choice is a spermicidal latex condom.

Condoms are referred to as skins, rubbers and natural membranes. Although most condoms are effective to prevent pregnancy, the natural skin and non-latex condoms are perforated with microscopic holes or membranes that allow STD viruses to pass through. Therefore, the only condom to use for safe sex is a latex condom.

If condoms fail to protect it is mostly the fault of the user because they have used them in a slipshod, or improper way. Therefore, you must be consistent and follow the guidelines described in this chapter.

Lubricants and Application

Throughout the following sections of the book we will be referring to lubricants. Lubricants come in two categories. The first category are lubricants that contain a spermicide known as Nonoxynol-9. The spermicides in this category are used as contraceptives because they eliminate the effect of the male sperm on the female egg. Some medical tests have revealed that spermicides, especially ones containing Nonoxynol-9, are effective in reducing the chance of infection from certain sexually transmitted diseases. The second category of lubricants come in a variety of consistencies (water-based, oil-based, scented, colored, unscented, clear, liquids, gels, flavored) and are used primarily to enhance pleasure, **not** to prevent pregnancy or disease.

Never use oil-based lubricants with a latex condom. Oil-base lubricants will destroy the integrity of the latex condom.—A broken condom is useless as protection.

When purchasing a lubricant, read the label and see what ingredients are listed. Make sure whether it is either an oil-based or a water-based product. Be aware of any active ingredients in the lubricant that you may be allergic to, as this will cause an irritation or a rash. Be wary of some of the new products coming on the market that are silicone based lubricants. These products are made with Dimethicone and do not have any protective value whatsoever.

Lubricants used with latex condoms can prevent the discomfort associated with dryness during intercourse and also make condoms less likely to break. Water-based lubricants, like KY jelly ®, and various spermicidal jellies, are strongly recommended.

Sexual intimacy does not necessarily mean only sexual intercourse. You can engage in sexual activity that would still involve risk regarding STDs. For example, you can contract a sexually transmitted disease by having anal sex or oral sex. Therefore, all the information that we discussed regarding safe sex applies to all forms of sexual intimacy.

In order to have oral sex you should always use a latex condom and in the case of oral sex on a woman you should use a dental dam or latex barrier. If necessary you can cut a male condom into a latex barrier and use it as a barrier when performing oral sex on a woman. It is always advisable to use a latex condom with spermicide and lubricant when performing anal sex.

CHAPTER V

Making Sex Safer

If you decide to be sexually active you must be honest and communicate with your partners and insist on practicing safer sex.

The only completely effective method of preventing sexually transmitted diseases and pregnancy is abstinence. For those unwilling to engage in abstinence, it's essential to practice safe sex.

Communicating with your partner about your concerns, fears, desires, and choices are essential to making sex safer. Do not be afraid to ask about your partner's health and sexual history. Honesty on your part communicates that you are and promotes honesty from your partner; you both can them make informed decisions. But remember—it's up to you to protect yourself in every sexual relationship. Don't depend exclusively on talking to protect yourself from STDs. Your partner may not realize, or reveal, things that could put you at risk for STDs. Together decide what you both feel comfortable doing sexually, and what precautions you will take. It is okay if you feel awkward or uncomfortable talking about sex. Sharing those feelings with your partner helps. Talking about sex can be easier if you are bale to talk about other personal and emotional issues. Being intimate is much more than a sexual act. If discussions about relationships, emotions, or sex are difficult for you, seek counseling from capable professionals who can help you learn some important skills in communication.

Safer Sex

Kissing, hugging body rubs while partially dressed, back rubs, foot rubs, caressing, nibbling at each other's bodies except for the genitals or anus, talking bout sexual fantasies, dry humping, showering together, licking or fondling your partners body except for the genitals or anus, giving an oil or lotion massage, stroking your partner, manual stimulation to your partner's sex organs as long as you have no cuts, abrasions or open sores. Preferable if you are going to have an orgasm you should use a condom whenever possible, rubbing your bodies together as long as there is not broken skin on your partner's body. Using your hands to masturbate each other making sure that you do not ejaculate in or near any of your partner's body orifices, or touching each other while sleeping together.

If you are going to do anything more than what is outlined above, you need to honestly communicate with your partner about the safe sex precautions.

The following are some ways to bring up the topic of safer sex with your partner before you get too involved.

You plan the moment. Do not wait until the middle of a passionate moment when your passions are running too fast and your hormones have taken over.

First, when you are by yourself—practice what you want to say because talking about safe sex sometimes makes people very embarrassed and nervous. Give yourself some time and try rehearsing. Pretend you are playing a role with your partner. Then try to find a private, comfortable, cozy place where you feel at ease and can talk privately with your partner. Here are some suggestions on how to start the conversation.

You could start off by saying "A lot of people are talking about using condoms and how they protect. I think it's a good idea. How do you feel?" If your partner is resistant and says something like, "I don't want to talk about it," or "forget it," or "I don't like condoms," you can say, "Why do you dislike condoms? Can't we give them a try? Do this for us."

Another approach would be if you're already involved, you could start off by saying "I don't want to give up sex but AIDS and pregnancy have me scared. I'm going to use condoms whenever I have sex." If your partner resists and says something like, "don't you trust me?" or "do you think I have a disease?" or "don't you think I know better?" you can respond by saying, "I do trust you but how can I be sure of your former partners or mine? Trust has nothing to do with pregnancy."

Another approach, "I have been thinking a lot lately about all the diseases that you can get when you have sex, but if we use condoms and spermicide we can prevent them." If your partner replies, "I don't like condoms, they're no fun," or "they destroy the spontaneity of sex." or "I think condoms are stupid" you can say, "Well, I will keep them with me and it could be fun if we put it on together. Let's give it a try because I want to do this or I need this." Try to put it on an equal level so that both people are agreeing and know that it is for the best for both people.

Another way is to propose "I'd love to make love with you, but I always use condoms to play it safe." If your partner is unsure or resists or says something like, "I think it's going to ruin the feeling for me," or "it's not macho to use condoms," you can reply, "it might feel a little different, but let's try it. After all, sex won't feel good at all if we never have it. We need to use condoms and a spermicide."

Plan ahead. If you feel you are going to have sexual contact make sure that you take along some spermicide and condoms. Don't depend on the other person. Play it safe. After the first several times you both will have a peace of mind and you'll find that having sex is more enjoyable when you feel safe and secure. Your partner may try to talk you out of it but remember that no sex, no matter how great you think it might be, is worth a lifetime of pain and suffering or even death. It is possible to become infected or pregnant if you have just one unprotected sex act.

CHAPTER VI

Sexual History

Good communication between partners is essential to make sex as safe as possible and to dramatically reduce the risk of contracting an STD.

It is hard to talk to your lover about sex, past sexual habits and medical history because at best most people are embarrassed and they will probably sound like they are judging or criticizing. There is also enormous cultural and religious barriers that keep men and women, for different reasons, from talking about sex with each other. Even our society makes it difficult for men and women to talk to each other about sex. Men are suppose to know everything about sex, it is not macho to discuss sex with a woman. Women, on the other hand, were brought up to believe that you are not a lady if you talk about sex. Responsible, caring adults must talk about sex and medical history before hand. Chapter Two thoroughly explains the methods about honest communication between partners.

Safe sex is not possible until both partners have had a medical exam and blood test and have tested negative for ALL sexually transmitted diseases and waited the appropriate incubation period to ensure a clean bill of health. During the waiting period both people must not engage in any sexual activity or IV drug use.

The partners should agree up front to practice safe sex using condoms and spermicidal until he exams are completed and both are free of any STD. Practicing safe sex by having a medical exam and blood test only relates to STD's and does not protect women from unwanted pregnancy.

If you feel that you do not know the person well enough to discuss such things, or do not feel comfortable to discuss these things with your partner, then you have to ask yourself the question, should you really be developing a sexual relationship with someone you cannot talk to about sex and your emotions.

Precautions You Should Take Regarding Sex

Learn to communicate effectively with your sexual partner.

Never mix alcohol or drugs with sexual activity: use humor and honesty instead.

Choose lower-risk sexual activities

Use latex barriers to prevent exchange of semen and vaginal secretions. Be sure you know how to use condoms correctly and understand their advantages and limitations. Learn about lubricants.

Remember that contraceptives other than condoms (including birth control pills, intrauterine devices, and diaphragms) do **NOT** protect you against STDs. To prevent both pregnancy and STDs, use a condom along with the other contraceptive methods. **Precautions cannot eliminate all risks, but you can make sex much safer.**

CHAPTER VII

Sexually Transmitted Diseases

Sexually Transmitted Diseases—What Are They?

STDs (Sexually Transmitted Diseases) sometimes called Venereal Diseases are infections you get from sexual contact with a person carrying the infection. More than 25 STDs have been currently identified.

Sexually transmitted diseases (STDs) are infections you transmit or receive during unprotected sexual contact. There are many: chlamydia, gonorrhea, genital herpes, and infection with HIV (the virus that can cause AIDS) are just a few. Some STDs spread more easily than others. You never become immune to STDS. You can get re-infected and you can have more than one STD at the same time. Some STDs show few or no symptoms: many people are infected and spread the microorganisms without knowing it.

One STD, hepatitis B, is preventable by vaccination. There is effective medical treatment for many other STDs, like chlamydia and gonorrhea. There is only limited therapy for viral STDs, like genital warts (which are caused by human papillomaviruses), herpes, and HIV infection.

STDs are at an epidemic rate in the United States today. They are among the nation's most common and contagious diseases, affecting at least 40 million Americans. It is estimated that there are about 12 million new cases per year.

Who is at Risk for STDs?

Any sexually active person is vulnerable to contracting a sexually transmitted disease. If you have unprotected sex the risk is greatly increased. No one is immune. It is estimated that 1 in every 6 adults in the United States has had or does have an STD. Even though many of these STDs are curable, many are not. Even among the more treatable ones, repeated infections can often toughen the virus responsible to the point where it becomes resistant to treatments and medications.

Please do not use this information in this section to self-diagnose or treat yourself. If you have any symptoms or suspect you have an STD, get medical care promptly and take the time to follow-up after your complete treatment to make sure you are cured.

Are There Warning Signs or Symptoms of STDs?

Most STDs have symptoms or warning signs of some sort. It's important to pay attention to any and all signals that your body sends you. However, sometimes the symptoms are so mild that they go unnoticed, especially in the case of women. Therefore, if you have had sex with someone who might have a STD, the only sure way to determine infection is a blood test and exam from a doctor or other medical professional.

Because STDs can effect anyone it is important to know what to look for in yourself and others. Be especially alert to body changes in the genital areas. Sometimes these warning signs might appear right away or they may not show up for weeks or even months. Sometimes the symptoms will not appear or they will appear and disappear; however the disease is probably still active. STDs do not go away by themselves, therefore do not be lulled into a sense of false security if the symptoms disappear. You must have proper medical treatment.

Risk Factors

Sexually transmitted diseases such as aids, syphilis, hepatitis, gonorrhea, venereal warts, chlamydia and herpes are no longer someone else's problems. STDs are now everyone's problem, including teenagers. Many infected people are symptom free and may unknowingly pass infections on to others. Even if you think your partner is not that kind of person who would have an STD, you can't be sure because when you sleep with someone, in a way you're sleeping with all of their past partners as well.

Personal Exam For Risk

You are not at risk for STDs if you're NOT sexually active and practice abstinence. You are probably not at risk if you have been in a long term relationship for ten years or more and neither you nor you partner has had other partners, received a blood transfusion or blood products, used IV drugs or has come in contact with an infected person through their occupation.

ASK YOURSELF THE FOLLOWING QUESTIONS TO DETERMINE WHETHER OR NOT YOU ARE AT RISK

1. How sure can I or my partner be that neither one of us is infected with AIDS or another STD?
2. How sure can I or my partner be that our past partners were not infected?
3. Have I been sexually active with more than one partner in the past ten years?
4. Is it possible that my partner has been exposed to IV drugs or received a transfusion of blood products since the late 1970's?

5. Can I become infected with STD by sleeping with an infected person only once?
6. Do I practice safe sex?
7, Did I discuss STDs and medical history with my partner before having sex?

STDs are a fact of life. If you are sexually active you're at risk regardless of your age, race, occupation or sexual preference. Furthermore, that risk is increasing because more and more people are getting STDs and new STDs are also being identified. The key to reducing your risk is to be informed about STDs and how to prevent them.

This book is not intended as a substitute for professional medical care or a thoughtful consideration of the personal medical risk involved in sexual expression today. If you suspect you have an STD, get medical care promptly. Control and safety are the major items regarding STDs. First you must learn about STDs. Second, you must recognize their symptoms and the body's warning signals. Third, you must get early and proper medical treatment, and fourth you must learn how to prevent STDs by practicing proper prevention techniques.

STDs
The following is not an all-inclusive list of STDs; however, the main ones are outlined for your assistance in this booklet. They are as follows: herpes, condyloma (venereal or genital warts), chlamydia, AIDS (acquired immune deficiency syndrome), gonorrhea, hepatitis, syphilis and vaginitis.

Symptoms
Recognizing symptoms is the most important way of controlling the spread of STDs. Symptoms are your body's way of telling you something is wrong. Be especially alert to changes in your body. When something

feels or looks different seek prompt medical care. If you are a woman you must be especially careful because sometimes early symptoms of an STD are noticeable in men but not in women. Frequently, a woman's first clue that she may have an STD is learning that a sex partner has one.

Most STDs can be cured if treated early. Women of childbearing age need to be particularly alert. STDs frequently cause problems with reproductive organs, making it difficult or impossible for a woman to get pregnant. In addition they're capable of causing diseases in newborns.

How Can I Get More Information?

You may obtain additional information about STDs by writing to the STDs Foundation, P.O. Box 511, Troy, Michigan 48099. Another phone resource is the VD National Hotline at 1-800-227-8922. In California call 1-800-982-5883 or the AIDS Hotline 1-800-342-AIDS.

Early Diagnosis

Early diagnosis gives a person the best chance for successfully treating an STDs. Even if a disease can't be cured, it can often be controlled. Here are some important things for a person to keep in mind if they've noticed any symptoms:

Eight Step Program

1. Be sure to be completely open with your doctor about what areas of your body have been bothering you.
2. If you have an STD then talking with your partner can be difficult. Ultimately though it is the most caring thing you can do and the only way to avoid becoming re-infected.
3. As soon as you are diagnosed, take a quiet private moment to discuss your treatment with your physician and then explain to your

partner(s) why they need an evaluation and possible treatment. Encourage you partner to seek treatment, too. Try not to pry into each other's past or place blame but be honest and show you care.

4. Make sure that you take the current medication prescribed by your physician and use the medication in the manner you are supposed to.

5. Go back to your doctor for a follow-up exam and tests according to his or her instructions.

6. Make sure you don't share your medications with someone else. Everyone should consult their own physician as to the proper medication and dosage.

7. Make sure you consult with your doctor to be reassured that you are cured or have the STD under control. Viruses are known for lying dormant and flaring up. The chance of this is increased if one hasn't gone through their whole prescribed treatment.

8. During your period of treatment you may be asked to abstain from sex or take other precautions. Consult with your doctor to find out when it is safe to have sex again. Don't have sex until you and your partner are completely cured.

Guide For STDs
This guide to STDs was prepared to help you better understand STDs, what they are, their symptoms, treatments and if they are life threatening. Knowing about and understanding STDs is the proper way to ensure a happy and healthy sexual future.

HERPES SIMPLEX VIRUS (HSV)
Herpes is actually a family of viruses that causes a variety of diseases that almost everyone comes into contact with. Examples of such ailments are chicken pox, mononucleosis and fever blisters. The herpes simplex virus or genital herpes usually affects the mouth or the genitals; it is the simplex

virus that is an STD. Over 40 million people have herpes. This viral infection is so widespread that support groups for people with herpes have formed in many cities. At present the infection has no cure and, understandably, many worry about herpes. Many people get only one outbreak while others must learn to control the infection.

Symptoms—The first episode usually occurs from 2 to 21 days after exposure. Symptoms may include swelling, pain, itching or burning at the site of the infection. This is followed by reddening and finally tiny blisters, which may then burst forming tender ulcers which crust and eventually heal. Some of the additional symptoms that may be experienced are fever, chills, lethargy, muscle aches or headaches. Some may have a burning or tingling feeling during urination or have a discharge of a liquid-like substance. Herpes sores come and go, but the virus remains. Symptoms begin with one or more fluid-filled blisters that open into sores. Sores may be painful and accompanied by swollen glands. Oral herpes produces sores around the mouth, genital herpes produces sores around the genitals and buttocks. The sores or blisters first open then heal as new skin tissue forms. During a first outbreak the area is usually painful and may itch, burn or tingle. Herpes may also infect the urethra, and urinating might cause a burning sensation. The first outbreak might last up to several weeks. When the sores are completely healed, the active phase of the infection is over. Symptoms may vary form one person to the next and in some people the first infection is so mild it goes unnoticed. Even so, subsequent re-occurrences of the disease could cause sores to reappear. Be aware that some people who have herpes have very minimal symptoms and do not seek medical treatment. Some people have frequent re-occurrences, while others have them rarely. Re-occurrences generally decrease as time goes on.

Treatment—Herpes can't be cured, but it can be controlled. Drugs called Acyclovir or Zovirax may speed healing and prevent re-occurrences. You can help, too. Keep herpes sores clean and dry, and don't scratch them. Pregnant women who have herpes should tell their doctors so that precautions (such as Cesarean delivery) can be taken to spare the baby from being infected.

Prevention—To prevent getting or spreading herpes, avoid sex during flare-ups and learn to recognize the sores. If you touch a herpes sore, wash your hands before touching your eyes, your mouth, or your partner. Use a condom between flare-ups. Reduce the stress in your life, too. Stress can trigger herpes outbreaks.

CONDYLOMA (VENEREAL WARTS)

Genital warts occur most often in young, healthy, sexually active men and women—especially in couples who don't use protective condoms for birth control. Without treatment, these warts cause cellular changes that could progress to genital cancer, especially in the cervixes of women. If you're pregnant, warts can be transmitted to your infant or block a normal delivery, so that a Cesarean (surgical) delivery may be needed. If you and your partner aren't both treated, you're likely to pass the virus back and forth to each other (the "Ping-Pong" effect).

Symptoms—Venereal warts can be flat or shaped like little cauliflower. They grow on the penis, vagina, and cervix and in and around the rectum and throat. The growths may take months after exposure to appear, and often they're so tiny they go unnoticed. Since they're hard to see, especially in the vagina or rectum, a thorough medical exam may be necessary to diagnose them.

Treatment—Venereal warts are more difficult to remove when they're bigger, so don't delay. They're usually removed with chemicals such as podophyllin (except on pregnant women). Sometimes warts are frozen off with liquid nitrogen or are surgically removed. Repeat treatments often are necessary to remove all warts. A single wart can multiply into many.

Prevention—To prevent venereal warts, use condoms, know your partner and get regular medical exams. Also, learn to manage stress—

outbreaks of venereal warts may be related to your stress level. Pregnant women should be especially cautious as babies can be infected with venereal warts during childbirth.

AIDS

AIDS is the deadliest STD. The virus destroys the body's immune system, making a person vulnerable to attack from thousands of other viruses. Many people who have the HIV virus don't have AIDS, but they can pass it on. High-risk groups include gay and bisexual men, people who share IV needles, and sex partners of these groups. AIDS is spread through exposure to infected blood or semen, not by casual contact.

Symptoms—Swollen lymph glands, fever, night sweats, severe fatigue and weight loss. Many AIDS symptoms are similar to those of other diseases except that AIDS symptoms persist and get worse. If you get sick often or if an illness lasts a long time, seek medical care right away. The AIDS virus attacks the body's immune system and leaves the person with AIDS unable to fight off many other kinds of infections and cancers.

Treatment—If you're experiencing AIDS symptoms, see a doctor immediately. Currently AIDS has no cure and no vaccine, but treatments are being tested. For information, call the AIDS 24-hour hotline at 1-800-342 AIDS or the Gay and Lesbian Crisis Line at 1-800-221-7044.

Prevention—If an infected partner's blood, semen or vaginal fluids enters your body through a break in the lining of the rectum, vagina, mouth or through a needle puncture, you can be infected with the virus. You may not know you have cuts or sores in these areas as they may not hurt or even be visible. Reduce your risk of getting AIDS by avoiding exposure to a partner's bodily fluids (blood or semen) by using a latex condom plus spermicide. Never share an IV needle under any circumstance. Do not allow body fluids to contact the skin.

GONORRHEA

Gonorrhea is so widespread, a new infection occurs every 12 seconds. If untreated, gonorrhea can cause sterility and, in women, pelvic inflammatory disease (PID.)

Symptoms—The incubation period for men is one day to two weeks and is generally longer for women (7 to 21 days). Men may notice a milky white pus discharge and painful or tingling urination. Women often have no early symptoms, but later they may develop a painful burning sensation during urination or a yellowish or whitish vaginal discharge. Left untreated, these symptoms may generate into abdominal pain, bleeding between periods, vomiting and fever. If left untreated, the real danger is that the infection will ascend into the seminal vesicles, the rpididymis or the prostate, potentially causing sterility. It can also cause a narrowing of the urethra, making urination permanently more difficult. In women the bacteria will invade the reproductive system, usually the ovaries and fallopian tubes, causing pelvic inflammatory disease. This can cause infertility. The bacteria in both men and women can sometimes get loose elsewhere inside the body and attack heart valves, the brain, joints or the blood stream. Pregnant women can pass the disease on to their babies during childbirth. Many states require infant's eyes to be treated with special silver nitrate or penicillin eye drops to prevent infections that can lead to blindness from gonorrhea.

Treatment—Gonorrhea is a bacterial infection and can be quickly cured with antibiotics. However, some gonorrhea germs are penicillin-resistant.

Prevention—The best protection against gonorrhea is to know your sex partner. If sexually active, learn the symptoms of the infection, use condoms and other precautions to reduce risk, and get regular medical checkups.

VAGINITIS

Vaginitis is really a group of diseases. The three most common are trichomonisas, yeast infection, and gardnerella. Although mainly a woman's problem, vaginitis can be carried and spread by men. In fact, trichomoniasis is often called "Ping-Pong" because sex partners don't know they have it and keep re-infecting one another. Some forms of vaginitis, such as yeast infections, also occur in women who are not sexually active.

Symptoms—The vaginitis disease all shares a common symptom discharge. Trichomoniasis produces a frothy, yellow discharge and causes persistent itching or burning. The discharge may have a unpleasant odor. Yeast infections produce a discharge that looks like cottage cheese and can cause an intense itch. Gardnerella causes a grayish-white, watery, strong-smelling discharge.

Treatment—Both you and your partner should be treated for trichomoniasis to avoid re-infecting each other. Trichomoniasis is treated with a medication called metronidazole. Yeast infections are treated with nystatin vaginal suppositories or creams. Gardnerella is treated with ampicillin or metronidazole. Be sure to take all the medication prescribed for you.

Prevention—Vaginitis can be difficult for a woman to prevent. These precautions will help to reduce the risk. Wash the vaginal area daily with soap and water, rinse, and pat dry. Don't us douches or strong deodorant soaps. They can upset the vagina's natural chemical balance, permitting the growth of yeast. Wear cotton or cotton-crotch undergarments. They provide better air circulation than other types of materials, which discourages infections.

SYPHILIS

Syphilis is caused by corkscrew-shaped bacteria. Unless treated, it can cause heart and brain damage, even death. Pregnant women can give the infection to unborn babies.

Symptoms—The first symptom of syphilis is a painless sore, which may not be noticeable. Later symptoms include rash and fever. Those symptoms disappear but, if untreated, the disease leads to serious damage years later.

Treatment—Syphilis is treated with antibiotics. Early treatment is important because although symptoms of the infection may disappear, the disease remains in the body and progresses to the next stage of severity.

Prevention—As with gonorrhea and other STDs, knowing your sex partner is the best prevention against syphilis. If sexually active, use condoms and other precautions and get regular medical exams.

CHLAMYDIA

Chlamydia is the fastest growing STD, especially among young people 15 to 25. It's already more widespread than gonorrhea. It may be overlooked because it's often symptomless and may not be tested for. In women it may not be noticed until its later and more serious stages. If untreated, chlamydia can cause sterility in both women and men.

Symptoms—Chlamydia can be like a time bomb. At first, it's symptomless, then complications flare up. When early symptoms do appear, they're often mild. These symptoms could take the form of an odorless discharge or burning. A complication in women is pelvic inflammatory disease (PID), a major cause of sterility and ectopic (tubal) pregnancy. PID symptoms include fever, pain during sex and abdominal pain.

Treatment—Men diagnosed with chlamydia should tell their partners right away. Often a woman doesn't have symptoms. She learns she has chlamydia only when a sex partner tells her he is infected. When diagnosed early, chlamydia can be cured easily with antibiotics. New tests for chlamydia are becoming more widely available.

Prevention—The best way to avoid chlamydia is to know your sex partner. If either of you had sex with anyone else, use precautions, especially condoms, and have regular medical checkups. A pregnant woman should be especially cautious because untreated chlamydia can cause eye, ear, or lung infections in her baby.

HEPATITIS

Hepatitis B mainly attacks young men and women in their teens and twenties. Like herpes, once you contract hepatitis, you become a carrier for life. Hepatitis B attacks the liver. Both hepatitis B virus (HBV) and hepatitis C (HCV) can be sexually transmitted, however, you *MUST* go way beyond normal prevention with hepatitis because it can be spread by direct contact with an infected person through open sores and cuts. If you know someone who is infected, you can contract hepatitis B by using the same glass, toothbrush, razor or using the same pierced jewelry as someone who has it. Once you have hepatitis B your chance of contracting liver cancer is much higher than normal.

Symptoms—Dark urine, unexplainable tiredness, nausea, symptoms like stomach flu or yellowing of the eyes and skin are all common symptoms. Consult your doctor right away if you experience any of these.

Treatment—The treatment for hepatitis B consists of a series of shots by a doctor, bed rest and a special diet high in protein and carbohydrates.

Prevention—Unlike other STDs, hepatitis B can be transmitted by direct contact with saliva. Therefore, you cannot kiss an infected person or come in contact with any open cuts or sores on the infected person's body. Using condoms and safe sex precautions will *NOT* prevent infection. When properly used, latex barriers and latex condoms with a spermicide will protect against infected semen and vaginal secretions, however, they will *NOT* protect you from becoming infected with hepatitis B. Hepatitis B is transmitted through direct contact with infected persons and is more infectious than other STDs.

What Should You Do If You Have A Sexually Transmitted Disease?

If you believe you have some of the symptoms of a sexually transmitted disease remember that this is a disease that can be treated. It is not a stigma. Do no become embarrassed or worried. Early diagnosis is the key to treatment and control. The first thing to do is to see your physician. Diagnosis is the first step in the treatment and cure for most of the diseases. Be sure to tell your doctor everything—your complete sexual history and partners with whom you have been involved. Follow the medical treatment completely and take proper precautions during your treatment until your doctor says it is permissible to resume sexual activity.

Caring, lasting relationships are built not only on having fun together but also on caring about each other's well being. If you have a STD, you and your partner can work together to solve a common health problem that belongs not just to you or your partner, but to both of you. When you take the 8 steps toward treatment, you are talking steps that show you care about each other.

You Can Control Sexually Transmitted Diseases

Misinformation or really unrealistic expectations about sex contribute to the spreading of STDs. The first stage of controlling STDs is to correct his misinformation and myths about how people transmit the diseases and next to remove anxiety from sexual encounters by knowing how to practice safer sex.

The only sure ways of not contacting STDs is by abstinence from sex or having a monogamous relationship with someone that has had a complete medical exam and blood test and you know is disease free.

Cardinal Rule

First—learn about STDs.
Second—Recognize their symptoms & warning signals
Third—get proper medical treatment
Fourth—Learn how to prevent and use safe sex

Leading Cause of Infertility

Although PID (Pelvic Inflammatory disease) is not listed as a sexually transmitted disease, it is the leading cause of infertility and affects more than one million women each year. More than 100,000 women each year become infertile as a result of PID, and a great many of the ectopic or tubal pregnancies are due to PID.

PID is a pelvic inflammatory disease (PID), an infection of the upper genital tract that can spread to the uterus, ovaries, fallopian tubes, or other related structures, often resulting in future infertility.

PID is marked by lower abdominal pain and abnormal vaginal discharge. Other symptoms may include fever, pain in the right upper abdomen. Fever, flu like symptoms, painful intercourse and irregular menstrual bleeding, however, the symptoms may be so minor that you are not aware of the illness and left untreated can seriously damage the reproductive organs.

Condoms will reduce the risk of PID (according to study at the University of Pittsburgh Medical Center). In fact inconsistent use of condoms or not using them 100% of the time actually doubled the risk of PID.

When used correctly and consistently, male latex condoms will prevent transmission of gonorrhea and partially protect against chlamydia infection.

Inconsistent use of barrier methods of contraception, particularly condoms, is really harmful. If you are going to use barrier methods, you better make sure that you are using them correctly and consistently.

Quick Reference Chart For Most Common STDs.

Any of these STDs can be transmitted through sexual contact (including vaginal and anal intercourse or oral sex) with an infected partner who may or may not have symptoms.

	What are the signs?	How is it treated?	Possible problems
Chlamydia	Men: Burning on urination and discharge from the penis. Women: Often no symptoms until PID begins. People often have no symptoms but are still infected and able to transmit chlamydia.	Infected persons and their sexual partners must be tested and/or treated with antibiotics. Curable.	PID and infertility in women, including an increased risk of ectopic (tubal) pregnancy. In men, infection of the prostate and epididymis.
Human Papillomavirus Infection (HPV) (including genital warts, Condylomas)	Warts appear as painless growths around the genitals in men and women. Potentially pre-cancerous cell changes and some types of warts are not visible to the naked eye. People who are infected but who don't have symptoms can still transmit the virus	For warts: cryotherapy, laser, or chemical treatment. For cervical changes: cryotherapy or laser. Women must have regular, follow pap smears to check for recurrences.	Some cell changes, especially the cervix, can be pre-cancerous. Recurrences are possible.
Herpes	Sores around mouth (cold sores), genital or anus, often with small painful blisters. Sores may be hidden or overlooked. Oral-genital sex when your partner has a cold sore will cause genital herpes. Some people also have flu like symptoms. Some people have no symptoms but are still infected and able to transmit the virus.	Infected persons should avoid anal, oral, and vaginal intercourse while sores persist. Acyclovir capsules or ointment may be helpful but will not cure herpes. Repeat outbreaks are common but occur at very variable intervals. Treatable but not curable.	May contribute to cervical cancer and problems in newborn babies.

Hepatitis B	Fatigue, nausea, and jaundice with dark urine; some people, however, experience no symptoms, or only mild ones.	Diagnosis requires lab tests. Treatment directed at relieving symptoms and maintaining nutrition. Completely preventative by hepatitis B vaccine.	Some people become chronic hepatitis B carriers, whether or not they continue to show symptoms of hepatitis B infection. In some cases, scarring of the liver, liver cancer, or, really death may occur.4
Gonorrhea	Men: burning on urination and discharge from penis; sometimes sore throat or diarrhea. Women: often no symptoms until PID begins. Some people have no symptoms but are still infected and able to transmit the gonorrhea bacteria, especially when gonorrhea occurs in the throat or rectum.	Infected persons and their sexual partners must be tested and treated with antibiotics. Curable.	In women, PID and fertility problems, including an increased risk of ectopic (tubal) pregnancy. In men, infection of the prostate or epididymis. In both, injection of the joints, skin, and bloodstream.
Syphilis	Painless ulcer (chancre) at point of contact, usually penile shaft, around vaginal opening, or anus. Secondary stage may include a rash, swollen lymph nodes.	Infected persons and their sexual partners must be tested and treated with antibiotics. Curable without long-term consequences only if treated early.	If untreated, may affect brain, heart, pregnancies, or even be fatal.
Human Immunodeficiency Virus (HIV) Infection/AIDS (Acquired Immune Deficiency Syndrome)	Most people infected with HIV may show no symptoms for many years but are still able to transmit HIV. See ACHA's pamphlet, "HIV Infection AIDS: What Everyone Should Know," for more information.	New medications may slow down the course of HIV infection and prevent many complications. If you are concerned, consult an experienced health care provider or counselor about HIV antibody testing and appropriate medical evaluations.	HIV causes a spectrum of conditions from mild symptoms to a severe immune deficiency state (AIDS); people with AIDS experience unusual, life-threatening infections, cancers, and neurological problems.

CHAPTER VIII

The Male Sexual Anatomy

The male and female sex organs (genitals) are in a constant state of development and change from the time of birth until our death. The sex organs are also the reproductive organs of the body. When a man and woman have sexual intercourse and the man has an orgasm, sperm comes through his penis into the woman's vagina. If the sperm comes in contact with an egg in the uterus, then the woman can conceive and become pregnant (sperm can leak out of the penis and into the vagina without a man having an orgasm). The reproductive system of both the male and female are very simple in design, yet very complex in how they function. It is the same reproductive system that creates the pleasure and gratification of a sexual relationship.

The male's sex organs (genitals) are the penis and the scrotum. The testicles, two separate oval shaped eggs that produce sperm, are located inside the scrotum. Males produce sperm in their testicles. When a male becomes aroused and sexually excited, the penis will become erect and very hard. When a man obtains his ejaculation or climax, it is called an orgasm.

The cone-shaped part of the penis, the glans, is very sensitive, as well as the back-side of the shaft of the penis.

The sexual Anatomy of a male Consists of:

Penis: This organ is outside the male body. It is the organ that a man urinates with. It is also the sexual organ that during intercourse penetrates the females vagina. The end of the penis is usually cone-shaped and is referred to as the glans.

Testicles: These are two separate oval-shaped eggs (balls) that produce sperm.

Scrotum: The container or pouch of skin that holds the testicles and allows the sperm to be produced.

Vas Deferens: This tube-like part enables the sperm to move from the epididymis and through the urethra to the ampulla.

Ampulla: The enlarged end of the vas deferens. The ampulla is the staging area where the semen is made up from different body fluids along with the sperm.

Prostate : The prostate is a gland that surrounds the neck of the bladder and the urethra. The function of the prostate gland is to produce a thin milky fluid that also mixes with sperm to help protect them during their travels.

Seminal Vesicle: A mucus-like fluid is produced by this bag-like structure. This fluid then mixes with sperm and helps keep the sperm healthy.

Cowper's Glands: Consists of two small round glands below the prostate gland. The purpose of these glands is to produce a mucous-like fluid that lubricates the end of the penis before intercourse and to help the transport and protection of the sperm.

Urethra:

The urethra extends from the bladder to the opening at the tip of the penis. This tube is what carries the urine or semen to the outside of the body.

Urinary Opening:

Refers to the end of the penis and the slit or opening that urine and semen come out of.

Sperm:

A sperm (spermatozoa) is a tiny egg that looks like a tadpole. It is this cell that joins with the female's egg to create a baby.

Semen:

During sexual intercourse, a fluid is ejected from the urinary opening. The semen fluid is made up of seminal vaginal fluid, prostate gland fluid, a small amount of Cowper's Gland fluid and sperm. During intercourse, it is the job of the semen to work it's way into a woman's uterus to come in contact with the woman's egg produced by the ovaries.

Erection:

The process where the penis changes from flaccid (soft) to engorge itself with blood and become hard and erect.

Ejaculation:

The process when semen comes out of the urinary opening of the penis.

Foreskin:

Refers to the area of loose skin around the glans penis and the upper shaft of the penis. If a male is not circumcised, foreskin will refer to the cover of skin over the glans penis.

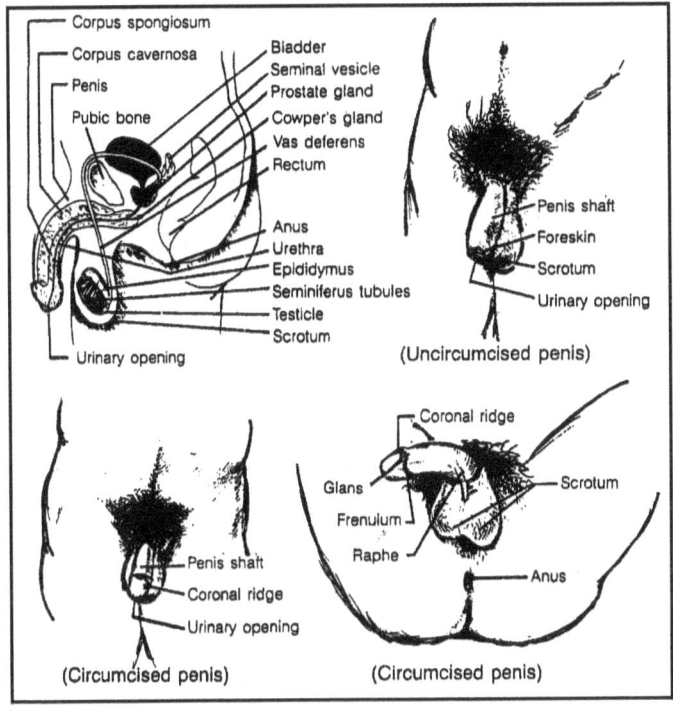

Male sex and reproductive system

The function of the penis is thought to be understood by most. However, "there is no organ about which more misinformation has been perpetuated," William Master, M.D., and Virginia Johnson of the Masters and Johnson Institute in Virginia once observed. "That amazing item of flesh has been venerated in cults, reviled and misrepresented in folk legends and mutilated, decorated, hidden, exposed, adorned and feared throughout the centuries. It is the item that is on every young man's mind as he grows up. It is the item that gives a great deal of frustration and anxiety because people are not sure how it should look, how it should perform, how they should treat it and how to properly use it."

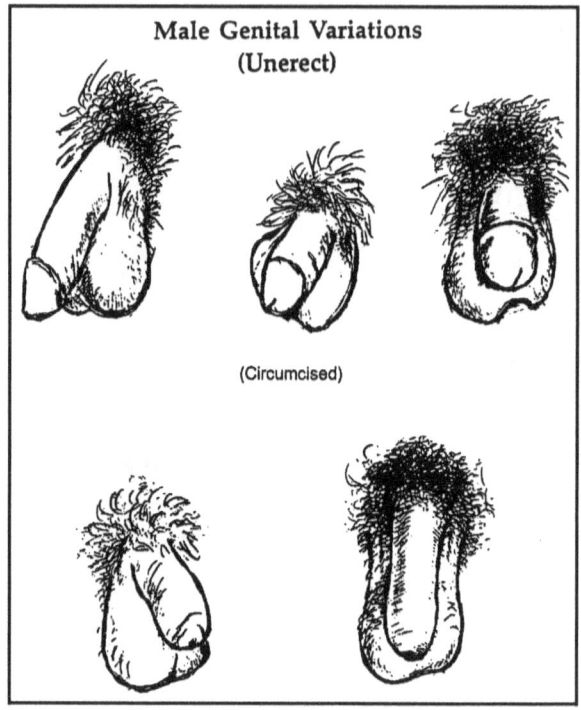

Cardinal Rule

Young men are caught up in the false big penis mythology and are always worried about how they measure up to others. However, the truth is that there is no correlation between penis size and sexual pleasure.

In truth, the reproductive cycle for the male is very simple. The male has two testicles. They are shaped like small eggs and held in the scrotum, a pouch of skin outside of the body. The purpose of the testicles is to produce the male eggs or cells which are called sperm. During intercourse, the sperm produced can enter into the female and fertilize the female's egg, eventually producing an embryo.

The process is initiated when the male becomes sexually aroused and excited. The male sperm that is produced in the testicles and has moved to the epididymis so that the sperm can grow and mature will leave the epididymis via the vas deferens and travel to the ampulla where it is combined with other fluids to create the semen. While this is happening, the Cowper's glands have produced a fluid to coat the urethra and protect the sperm as it travels through the penis. At this point, there is a great deal of pelvic thrusting and ejaculation whereby the semen is pushed through the urinary opening. The rhythmic contractions of the muscles near the base of the penis drive the semen to go like spurts. The actual amount of volume during ejaculation varies from man to man. It also tends to decrease with age and increase with the length of time between ejaculations. Ejaculation usually produces a tremendous sensation of release because after it occurs, there is a release of the muscle tension and a gradual relaxation of the penis. After an ejaculation, the man will then return to what is known as the refractory period between ejaculations. This term refers to the time that is necessary for the body to rest and recuperate before the male can perform an erection and orgasm again. The refractory period usually gets longer as you get older. However, the periods vary from man to man and the more frequently a man ejaculates, the shorter the in between period it is likely to be. However, the average male will only have an ejaculation orgasm once a day in a 24 hour cycle.

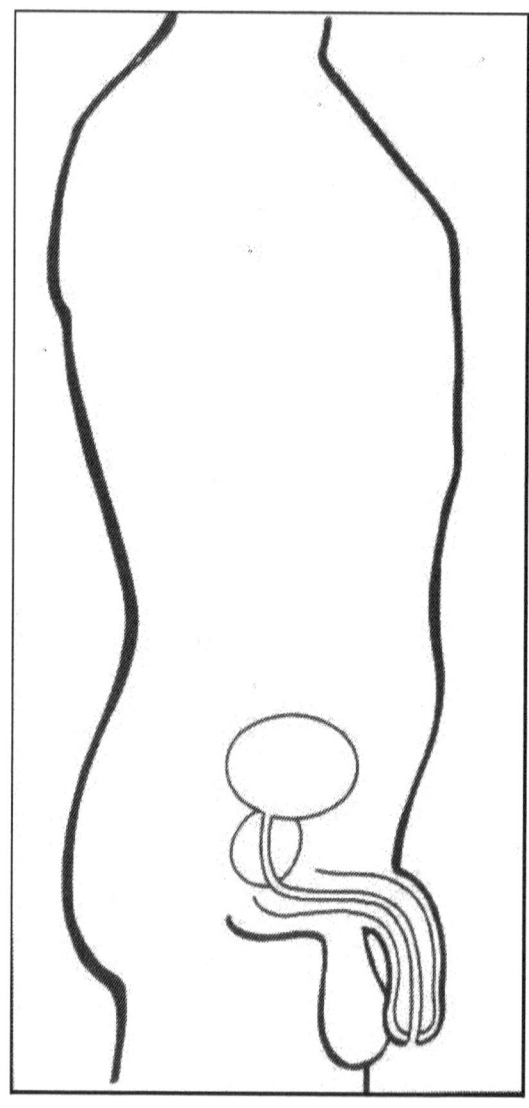

CHAPTER IX

The Female Sexual Anatomy

The female sexual organs are both inside and outside of the body and are more complex and thus there is frequently confusion or misunderstanding by both men and women regarding the female organs.

A woman should get a more accurate picture of her body. It is smart to know and understand how the body works and functions. If you have not had the opportunity before, take the time to give yourself a self- examination and explore the genital area.

The sexual area between a woman's legs is called the genital area or vulva. The woman has folds of flesh called lips in the genital area. The large outer lips are referred to as the labia majora or simply as the labia. Inside that is the labia minora, the small inner lips that protect the vagina opening. At the top of the small lips is a little bud referred to as the clitoris. The clitoris is extremely sensitive and when stimulated gives a woman sexual pleasure. When a woman is aroused, the blood vessels in the genital area and inner lips swell and her clitoris becomes erect. During an orgasm women will have a series of muscle contractions leading to an eventual release of tension.

The organs inside the woman are the vagina, uterus, fallopian tubes and ovaries.

THE FEMALE ANATOMY:

Vulva or genital area: That part of the external part of the female anatomy between her legs.

Mons veneris: The layer of fatty tissue that pads the pelvic bone underneath it. It is usually covered with hair.

Clitoral Hood: The clitoral hood may cover all of the clitoris or just a section. It is a layer of skin.

Clitoris: This is a very sensitive organ responsible for generating sexual excitement in a woman. It is very small, and when it is touched or aroused it will become enlarged with blood much like a man's penis and become erect.

Vaginal Opening: The vaginal opening refers to the area where the female's menstrual flow during her period flows out. It is also the opening where a erect penis penetrates during the act of intercourse.

Urethra Opening: The female urethra urinates from this opening.

Hymen: Refers to a piece of skin that is either partially or totally covers the vagina opening. It is believed that this delicate membrane can tell whether a person is a virgin or not. In reality, the hymen can become torn during any number of activities, including exercise and masturbation. Even doctors cannot tell for sure if a female has had sex. However, it is kind of a folklore that if the hymen is in place that a woman is still a virgin. However, medical reports have shown that because the hymen may be stronger in certain females, that even pregnant females can still have a hymen intact.

| Labia Minora: | Refers to the small inner lips that protect the vagina opening. |
| Labia Majora: | Refers to the large outer lips that protect the vagina area. |

Female External Genitals

Ovarian Follicles:	Refers to the compartments that make up the ovaries and that hold the individual ovum until it is ripe and ready to be released.
Ovaries:	Refers to the two oval shaped structures that holds the female eggs.
Ovum:	Refers to the tiny eggs that carries the mother's genetic matrix and that becomes fertilized during intercourse by the male's sperm.
Fallopian Tubes:	Refers to the fragile thin tubes that carry the ova to the uterus.
Uterus:	A pear shaped hollow muscular organ where the fetus will develop. It is this area that becomes blood enriched during the menstrual cycle and then sheds the enriched tissue during menstruation.
Fimbria:	Refers to the small finger-like extensions at the end of the fallopian tubes.
Cervix:	This a small opening between the uterus and the vagina. It separates the vagina from the uterus.
Bartholin's Glands:	Refers to the two small glands that are located inside the walls of the vagina and that have the capability to secrete fluid.
Endometrium:	This refers to the layer of skin on the uterus that gets thick and falls off during menstruation.

Vagina: Refers to the hollow passage way that connects the
                        uterus to the outside of the body and at the vagi-
                        na opening is the area where the small inner lips,
                        large inner lips and the clitoris are located.

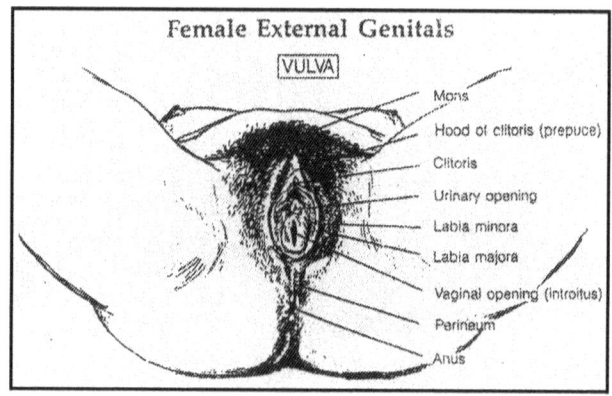

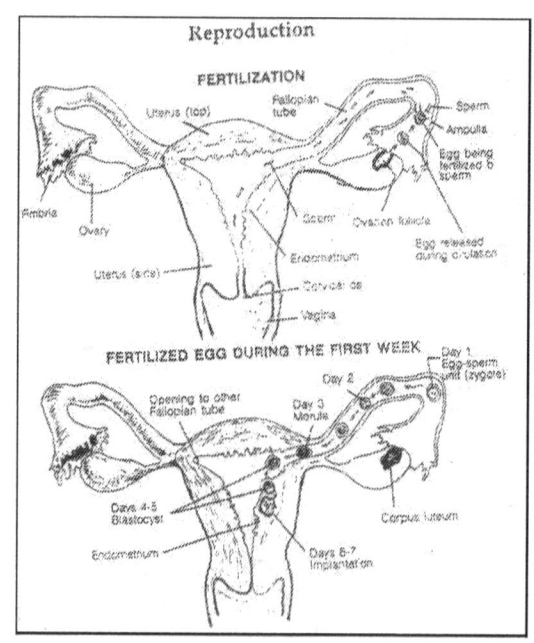

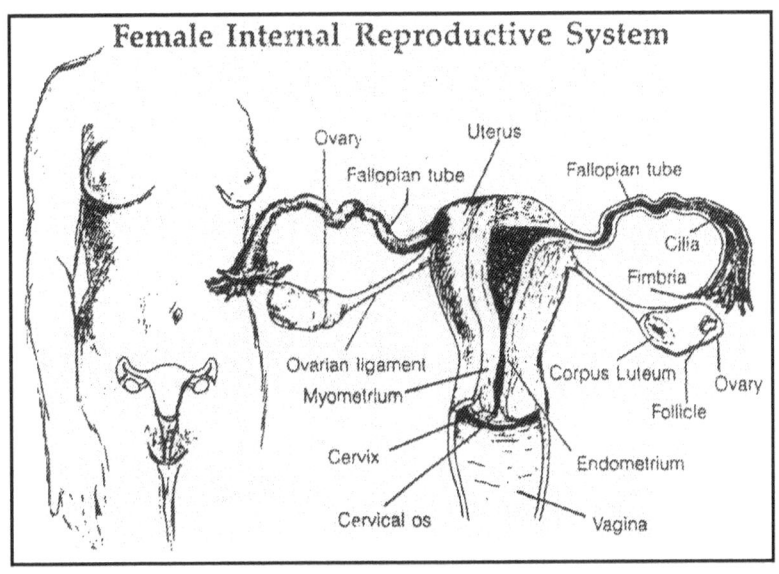

Female Internal Reproductive System

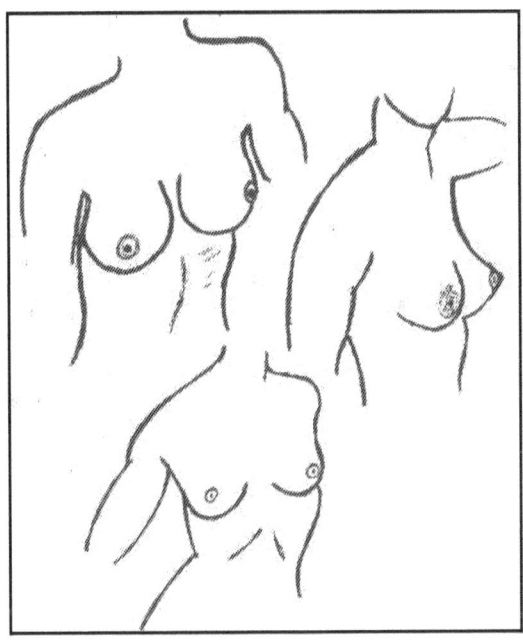

CHAPTER X

Beyond Safe Sex

By providing you with the following information and knowledge on safe sex and birth control, I hope you will fee secure and capable of taking control of your sexual activity and able to enjoy the pleasures of a good sexual relationship.

Birth control refers to many different methods that are employed to prevent unwanted pregnancies. However, birth control devices, technique and methods should never be confused with safe sex procedures because most birth control methods offer little or no protection regarding sexually transmitted diseases.

There are numerous birth control methods that are improper and non-effective. It is unfortunate because of the veil of secrecy that all too many people have been shocked when they found out that the woman was pregnant because they were under the false belief that they were practicing some form of birth control. All birth control devices either destroy or prevent the live sperm from performing its mission to fertilize the female egg. The average sperm has a life span of approximately 72 hours although some can live longer. The egg usually has a lifespan of approximately 24 hours during each monthly cycle. However, sperm stubbornly resist any effort to stop their progress and once the sperm reaches the cervix and starts its migration upward towards the fallopian tubes it may be there several days waiting for the egg. That is why many times people using different birth control methods are caught off guard.

The following are poor means of birth control:

The rhythm method depends on the people precisely knowing when ovulation takes place and avoiding having intercourse during this time. In theory it sounds fine. In actual practice many times it does not work because it is extremely difficult to predict with accuracy when ovulation is taking place.

Coitalus interruptus refers to the technique of withdrawing the penis from the vagina before the male ejaculation. This might seem a good technique, however, it is quite ineffective. Although this method requires no equipment or medication, it does not work very well for a variety of reasons. First, it requires the man to withdraw at the moment of greatest passion. It puts all the responsibility on the man but the consequences on the woman. Most importantly, in many cases, during sexual arousement, long before ejaculation occurs, tiny droplets of clear fluid filled with sperm escape from the tip of the penis. It takes only one sperm to cause conception.

— Female condoms are devices that are more expensive than male condoms. They have a greater tendency to be pushed aside or slip during intercourse and are not as reliable as the male condom.

— IUDs (Intra Uterine Devices IUD was effective as a birth control, 1% of the times when women did get pregnant there was a much higher chance the pregnancy would be ectopic (a pregnancy where the baby grows outside the uterus, usually in the fallopian tube). The major advantage of the IUD is it is a long- term birth control method and is very effective.) and in theory are great. A doctor must insert a small plastic apparatus into the uterus. As long as it remains in place, it will prevent pregnancies. However, in real life it turned out that the IUDs had many side effects. They had a tendency to cause bad pelvic infections. They were, at times, causing pain and undue cramping in the women.

Various Birth Control Methods

Today women have a wide variety of birth control options. The Norplant implant is a long-range and expensive method. There are female diaphragms, the cervical cap, the female sponge, numerous spermicides, jellies and creams designed to kill or immobilize sperm and are readily available. There's even a morning after pill when all else has failed or been forgotten. The morning after pill requires a prescription and a visit to the doctor's office.

— Sterilization is the ultimate birth control. Either the male or female is sterilized. This can be accomplished in one of two ways, either by a surgical procedure performed by a qualified physician or through the use of certain drugs.

— Oral contraceptives work and are effective as long as the woman remembers to take the pill. The chemical in the pill simply fools the woman's body into believing that she is pregnant so the ovaries will not release any eggs into the fallopian tubes. The hormones that are produced by the pituitary gland at the base of the brain control the growth of a few eggs each month and the production of the female sex hormone estrogen by the ovary. This process is fairly dependable, however, some women do have side effects from the use of the pill. Although there are many versions of the pill they still function in pretty much the same way. The pill can also be expensive in comparison to other forms of birth control. Since the pill relies upon the use of drugs in some cases the side effects can be severe and in a few cases it has been known to increase the risk of cancer in the ovaries. There are new formulas and pills coming on the market that have been tested and proclaim that they have eliminated the bad side effects. However, the choice of the pill should be left up to the woman and her physician if it is appropriate and effective.

— The latex condom is perhaps the easiest, most reliable and effective form of birth control if used properly with a spermicide. The medical statistics show that latex condoms are about 97% effective in preventing pregnancy. In addition, unlike all of the other previously mentioned methods or devices of birth control, it has one major advantage. It is an effective protection or defense against sexually transmitted diseases as well as unwanted pregnancies. Also, the condom is easily obtainable and transportable. This makes the condom the all around most versatile and effective form of safe sex and birth control.

Personal hygiene and personal exam

This section would not be complete without a discussion on personal hygiene and personal examination. Each of us should be responsible for doing self examinations regularly while bathing and notice any changes or symptoms in our bodies. This is very important for everyone, not just sexually active people.

Just below the vaginal opening and where the labia meet is a small area of smooth, usually hairless, skin. Below that is the anus (this opening is the area where fecal matter passes from the bowels). Women should always be careful to wipe from the front to the back after using the toilet to avoid having fecal matter transferred near the vaginal and urinary openings. This can be a common cause of vaginal and uterine infections.

Female Sexual Hygiene

Women, because of their special internal reproductive anatomy should pay special attention to their menstrual cycle. Physicians recommend that from the age of puberty you should keep a record of when you have your menstrual cycle. It can be invaluable for diagnosing many different types of problems and is much more accurate then vague recollections when you are talking to a doctor about changes in your cycle. The average length between one menstrual flow and the next is 28 days. However, cycle lengths vary from one woman to another. As a woman goes from puberty to menopause she can have tremendous variations in her cycle and amount of menstrual flow. Sometimes while a woman is maturing the periods may vary in timing, amount and color. All of this can be natural and should not be alarming. However, it is important to be aware of your menstrual cycle when you are discussing problems with your physician. The changes may be symptoms of something that needs treatment.

The female external genitals should be periodically examined. If any change takes place, you should contact your physician immediately. Just below the clitoris is a very small urinary opening. Below that is the vaginal opening. Because these openings are so close to each other, many women experience urinary infections after having sex. Women should understand their anatomy and learn to recognize signs of problems early, especially during the reproductive cycle.

Male Sexual Hygiene

A recommended routine for a man while in the shower is a self exam on his penis and testicles to see if there are any unusual marks, lumps, or coloring of the skin. If any change takes place, you should contact your doctor immediately.

Every man and woman must take responsibility for monitoring their own health and also be aware of the symptoms of sexually transmitted diseases. Always schedule a medical examination whenever changes or symptoms of a problem are noticed. Sexually active people should be checked twice a year for STDs and sexually active women should have a yearly pelvic exam and pap smear.

Unfortunately, many parents think that because teens look fine and are young adults, that regular check ups are no longer necessary. However, teens do need to have regular exams so that doctors can follow their growth and physical development and screen for changes that signal that something is not right or for disorders or substance abuse. It can be a great comfort to a teen if they have an established relationship with a doctor because it is very difficult for a teen to talk about sex, STDs and the private parts of their body. Embarrassment, fear or guilt cause a lot of teens to go untreated when they become infected with a STD. That is why even though the cure is available many go untreated and put a whole generation of teens at risk. It is estimated that 1 out of every 6 teens will contract an STD disease. Because most teenagers are very afraid of how their parents will react, they will go untreated.

In order to create a solid relationship between parent and teen and between two partners, you must have a free flow of communication. You may have empathy for the other person, however, we all know that it does no good to say to a loved one after the fact, "If I had only known."

Stay Healthy

Keep yourself physically fit and sexually active and you can go on enjoying satisfying and pleasurable sex almost to the very end of your life. A 72-year old woman told researchers Bernard Starr, Ph.D., and Marcella Weintar, Ph.D., "Our sex is so much more relaxed I know my body better, and we know each other better. Sex is unhurried and the <u>best</u> in our lives."

Tips to stay healthy*

- ✗ Eat a balanced diet
- ✗ Get plenty of rest
- ✗ Exercise regularly
- ✗ Avoid infections
- ✗ Learn to relax and deal with stress

✗ Do not take unnecessary medications—especially antibiotics and steroids

✗ Practice safe sex

✗ Do not use drugs like marijuana, speed, cocaine, downers, nicotine or heroin

*Department of Health and Human Services.

Cardinal Rule

A healthy body increases the pleasure of sex, sexual activity, can rejuvenate the body, and you alone have control over one of the greatest ways to pleasure yourself. Use this control wisely and prudently

Author Background

Rescue 911 Series Foundation

P.O. Box 511

Troy, Michigan 48099

Free information brochure: 877-473-9435

Phone line 877-4SEX HELP

Ronald A. Hagen is a highly motivated, investigative researcher with over 12 years of experience compiling information regarding sex, love and relationships.

Mr. Hagen was trained as an analyst and researcher while he was an agent with the Central Intelligence Agency. He has adapted this skill to the field of love and relationships, and has spent thousand of hours reviewing facts and theories about relationships. He has exhaustively examined hundreds of exit interviews of couples, has been involved with numerous support groups, and has corresponded with both the federal and state health departments on STDs and relationships. As a result of these experiences, Hagen has been exposed to virtually every theory regarding relationships.

Additionally, Mr. Hagen has worked with several school organizations in developing programs for teens. He is cochairman of the STDs foundation and has worked with the Michigan State Health Department to co-produce television programs for channel 62 regarding teen dating and safe sex. He has written brochures and pamphlets regarding safe sex and abstinence and was featured on cable TV in a half-hour program dealing with communication and components for developing a successful relationship.

He has appeared on the radio station WNZK for the program Bright Side of Aging in discussions regarding seniors and their evolving relationships.

Mr. Hagen has conducted seminars and lectures for numerous community organizations. He is the author of What You Always Wanted to Know About Sexually Transmitted Diseases, "The New Teen Dating Game, and Love, Sex and Relationships Where Would We Be Without Them. Hagen teaches courses at Macomb Community College regarding relationships and teen dating.

0-595-20995-5